HEALTH CARE

OBSERVATIONS

THAT YOU SHOULD KNOW!

BELEN F. CANTILLER

HEALTH CARE

OBSERVATIONS

THAT YOU SHOULD KNOW!

BELEN F. CANTILLER

To order additional copies of this book, contact:
Xlibris
1-888-795-4274
www.Xlibris.com
Orders@Xlibris.com
536525

PREFACE

As a health-care professional, a licensed registered nurse, I have gained and benefited from the many and various experiences I had in the health-care industry.

In this time of advancing technology of Facebook, Twitter, cell phones, computers, internet, website, satellite, information about any and everything abounds and surrounds us. Yet even if there is much that is known, the unknown seems infinite. What secret has everlasting life?

This book provides a slight insight of some of my medical experiences. Almost everyone is seriously concerned about having good health. I hope some of the observations, awareness from my listening, and some prudent advice I have gained maybe informative, interesting, and beneficial to you as readers of this book.

This is an insight of some of my experiences. It is a significant amount of involved observing and listening. As with all health-care situations, I have spent a great deal of time analyzing my own participation to determine how to improve the delivery and execution of my service.

While I am enormously proud of what I have accomplished, and I'm pleased of some of my practices and lessons learned. I know there is still more work to be done; I also recognize that I am not alone in this endeavor. With the help of others, we will close the gap of the healthcare divide.

This book details some of the inter reactions and relations among patients, family, healthcare professionals, workers, and others in a healthcare environment. It may be an antidote to the plague of chatter in this time of endless information.

BELEN F. CANTILLER

INSIGHTS, INCIDENTS, AND OBSERVATIONS OF A HEALTH-CARE PROFESSIONAL

"It is recommended to introduce to infants and toddlers to vegetables before fruits," Dr. Vivian Barrera said.

The idea is to have their taste buds, at an early age, enjoy vegetables.

"Do you wonder why they suck their thumbs?" Brenda said. "I tried some of the baby vegetable food. I have figured out."

BEFORE THESE INFANTS AND TODDLERS DEVELOP THEIR OWN EATING HABITS, IT IS RECOMENDED FOR THEM TO READ LABELS.

"A HEALTHIER YOU IS A DIVIDEND INTO EVERY FACET OF YOUR LIFE! The preventative benefits to keep you and your family healthy-when you eat almost right and right, you will feel 120% right," Bella said.

"If you can't stick with your diet, your doctor doesn't understand. Start taking the right kind-you know, a natural solution. That is why we focus on what you eat," Uncle Tet said.

"Cheer! Don't miss out opportunity to vastly improve your health," Auntie Puring said. "Just two more chances for us to be right!"

"It is healthier to question the obstacle with diet—which contributes to the obstacle—than to question with drugs that carry side effects," Uncle Tauro, said.

"Eating Western Diet and High Sugar Junk Food sets people up for disaster straight to the edge of a cliff," Baden said.

"People consuming traditional unprocessed foods-Cancer, Heart Disease, and Diabetes are found to be low.

"Eating Western diet increases in number of obesity and diabetes," Bebe Marlu said, "We still have more answers than questions."

"Stop coping with the ubiquitous junk and greasy food." *"Good chance you will return to normal."* Bi said.

Meg said, "Watch those bread it is one of the greatest sources of salt."

"Limit your salt to 1,500 milligrams a day," Jared said. "If more, it's salty!"

"A teaspoon of salt contains approximately 2,300 mg of sodium," Jovian said.

"Potassium is not stored in our body. Much is lost in perspiration. As you consume potassium you excrete sodium, keeping your blood pressure down," according to Von.

"Animal protein can harm the kidneys," Joshua said.
"Protein from plant sources is the surefire way."

"Vitamin C degrades in fruits and vegetables as it ages. Eat fresh produce soon after you buy it," Karl Manuel said.

"Have a daily dose of omega 3-s. Include 3-ounce servings of salmon, lake trout, herring, or other fatty fish a week," Nene said.

Shem said, "I eat cereal fortified with vitamin D that fend off my blues."

"Women should aim to get 46 G of protein while men should aim 56 G of protein daily. Some sources are from eggs, beans, and fish," according to Bethany.

"The daily recommendation of fiber intake is 25 G per day," said Jershon Jeiel.

"Why wheat make some people sick?" Manny asked.
"So the culprit is the wheat itself.
So here is the answer, Bess said, SKIP IT."

"I eat *oat meal* a powerfood with healthful benefits," said Ben. It has a low GI 152 per ¼ cup dry oats. It has a high level of protein, folate, manganese, fiber, copper, iron, phosphorous and vitamin B1. Eating whole grains lowers total cholesterol and LDL. Reduces risk of cardiovascular disease can lower risk of high blood pressure and type 2 diabetes. High fiber in oats stabilize blood sugar levels. It boost defenses of the immune system against bacteria, fungi, parasites and virus.
"Eating oatmeal gives you more energy. The bulk of the oatmeal make the stomach feel full longer and less hunger

for long time." Ben said, "*It is one of the healthiest breakfast choices.*"

"Some of us are genetically predisposed to high cholesterol levels. Diet is one of the key factors in raising and lowering cholesterol levels," Juvy said.

Lolit asked, "What are you going to have for breakfast?" Cami answered, "I don't know yet," Wanting to calculate calories and fat first.

"If a recipe calls for one to two eggs," Sing said, "Add a little teaspoon of water."

"What are the two problems with the eggs?" Cano asked? Raffy answered, "The yolk and the white."

"Are you hooked up on scrambled, fried, and hard-boiled eggs?"

Rose replied, "Leave them out."

Bessie said, "One large egg has about 186 mg of cholesterol. "How many eggs should you eat a week?

"Six but four eggs if you have high cholesterol, diabetes, and other heart condition. All B vitamins are found in eggs, B1, B2, B3, B5, B6, B12, choline, biotin, and folic acid. Eggs are good source of high quality protein. It has mineral, selenium, and iodine.

"Per hen can lay 200-300 eggs per year. Try brushing eggshells with lemon juice before adding water to the pot. It helps the shells from cracking and easier to peel. It is easy to cook and delicious."

"Extra-Virgin Oil each day-2 tbsp can be beneficial to your health. It contain substances called oleocanthol that inhibits inflammation by protecting against virus in the body. It is the highest monounsaturated fat among plant oils. It helps lower risk of developing heart disease by lowering LDL and increasing HDL. Helps prevent stroke. If consumed regularly it helps lower blood pressure both systolic and diastolic. It benefits insulin levels and blood sugar control for type 2 diabetes. Among menopausal women production of estrogen decrease calcium levels that weakens bone structures that affects hips, ribs and wrists. Olive oil helps calcium absorption and in preventing onset of osteoporosis. It helps protect the skin against the sun's effect of UV rays," according to Britta.

"FYI, Don't add olive oil to junk foods to make it healthy."

"I am allergic to hydrogenated oil," Maria Merle Lim said. *"Heavenly Longevity Gift."*

"The old standby condiments are still good. Ketchup, mustard, black pepper, hot sauce, salsa, relish, pickles, olive oil and vinegar." Auntie Pacing said, *"Just don't look for the preservative and coloring!"*

"Shhhhhhh . . . Beans are near-perfect health food. Low in cholesterol and fat, high in fiber, iron, folic acid, and good sources of protein. Your body and mind will be supercharged for hours. Discard the soaking water before cooking. Some mineral is lost, but you are getting rid 80% of the oligosaccharides that cause the flatulence."

"Frankly, my dear, I don't give a damn."

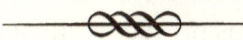

"Peanuts has low GI of 14. It contains more protein and vitamin A than any other nuts. It contains fiber, vitamin E, magnesium, manganese, vitamin B3(niacin), the most folate of any nuts, copper, phosphorous, potassium, phytosterol, resveratrol, and healthy fats.

"When eaten early in the morning peanuts and peanut butter helps decrease blood spikes and keep blood sugar levels more even throughout the day. Snacking peanuts and peanut butter two to three serving lowers LDL, triglycerides and increases HDL level because of their copper contents and keep you feeling full longer. Frequent peanut eaters had lower BMI and lowers risk of weight gain.

"Contains very high level of arginine, which causes the body to release more insulin and keep blood sugar more stable after eating carbohydrates.

"Vitamin A found in peanuts promotes the production of nitric oxide - a vasodilator that leads to the lower blood pressure. Vitamin E proven to protect skin from ultraviolet radiation and premature aging. It promotes clear skin. Good source of protein that is essential for growth and development. Boost memory power and normal brain functioning due to vitamin B3(niacin). Helps protect against degenerative diseases and cancer by inhibiting tumor growth," according to Baden.

"What is your preference peanut or peanut butter?"

"Soybean is super legume contains folate, vitamin A, vitamin K, calcium, magnesium, potassium, iron and high in protein. Also consider fermented versions like tempeh, fermented tofu, and soy miso. Same weight soybean contain more proteins and iron than meat, more calcium than cow's milk, more vitamin B1, vitamin B2, vitamin B6 than chicken eggs," according to Jershon Jeiel.

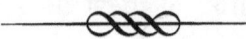

"People around the world are going banana with *avocados* and partly they are good for you! There are oodles of healthy options. Avocados contain vitamins C, vitamin E, vitamin K, and vitamin B6, high amount of fiber, iron, potassium, protein and loads of monounsaturated fat heart—healthy fats.

It prevents dry skin, brittle hair and nails. Repair damaged hair. Moisturize dry skin. Minimize wrinkles. They keep the skin youthful. Treat sunburns. Avocado is a rich source of glutathione, a detoxifying compound that helps break down carcinogens and free radicals. Vitamin C helps the body boosts the immune system against infectious agents, reduce cough and colds. Helps lower blood cholesterol, triglyceride levels, and fights anemia, as best as I know," Ann said.

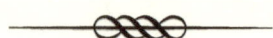

"Half a cup daily is sufficient for the highest rating among fruits," Nicah said, "GO BERRIES."

"Strawberries contains slow release carbohydrates, antioxidant (protects chronic diseases associated with aging) and all other berries blueberries, cranberries, blackberries, raspberries, are the best kind to optimize diabetes control. Source of vitamin A, vitamin C, vitamin E, B-complex group of vitamins. One serving of strawberries packs more vitamin C than an orange. The B-complex vitamin are needed for healthy skin, eyes, hair, and liver. They also help nervous system function regularly. There is 11 grams of carbohydrates in 1 cup. Strawberries can help control weight and weight loss. May help ward off wrinkles by promoting collagen synthesis and production. An anti-inflamatory benefits when strawberries are consumed three times a week. It has a natural tooth-whitener(strawberries contains malic acid), an enzyme found in some whitening toothpaste," according to Vanessa Barrera-Bales.

"Pour water in the basin add vinegar and stir. Wash your fruits and the water will be dirty. It will wash chemicals pesticides wax and dirt. Berries will keep them from molding and strawberries will last for weeks but eat your berries sooner to get the health benefit.

What's your favorite way to eat strawberries?"

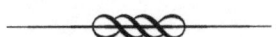

"Cranberries has low GI 23 calories in one cup. The fruit is initially white but turns a deep red when fully ripe. It is edible with an acidic taste. Most cranberries are processed into products such as jam, juice, sauce and dried. Cranberries served as a traditional accompaniment to turkey in Thanksgiving. Wisconsin is the largest producer and the second is Massachusetts in United States. Rich in fiber, manganese, and vitamin C. Contains tannin substances that act as natural antibacterial agent to fight urinary tract infection. Inhibits cancerous tumor and lower LDL cholesterol.

"Excessive amounts can cause upset stomach and diarrhea, as best as I know," Karl said.

"*Mangoes* deserve some spotlight as the national fruit of the Philippines, India and Pakistan," Tantan said. "It is the national tree of Bagladesh. When ripe it is sweet juicy delicate and has a distinctive flavor. It is rich in vitamin A, vitamin C, calcium, phosphorous, and fiber. Rich in minerals, copper, manganese, and zinc for production of red blood cells in the body. Rich in potassium helps control heart rate and blood pressure. It lowers the cholesterol level. It promotes good eyesight due to high content of vitamin A. It's vitamin C helps the skin clears the clogged pores, eliminate pimples, looking young and vibrant. Aids in reducing body fat and control blood sugar. It protects against leukemia, breast, prostate and colon cancer. The fiber in mangoes helps in digestion and elimination.

"Mangoes may be eaten raw mixed with salt or vinegar. It is widely used in cuisine, juices, smoothies, ice cream, fruit bars, pies, and as dried mangoes.

"Mangoes tops in taste if you get the right one. The fruit will have the best flavor if allowed to ripen on the tree. It is nutritious and delicious ending to a meal!

"The sugar content of less than 75% than the regular mangoes researchers are studying and anticipating to produce. *Stay tuned for updates!*"

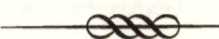

"A garden with a fruit bearing *guava* tree is opulence, Brenda said. It has 112 calories per one cup of guava chunks and 15 gm of sugar. When guava becomes yellow green to yellow and very aromatic then it is ready for consumption. The pink guava contains twice the amount of lycopene present in tomatoes. Lycopene protects the skin from UV rays and works against prostate cancer. It has four more times vitamin C content than oranges. High in vitamin C helps the body develop resistance against infectious agents and scavenge free radicals. Though guava don't contain iodine they are beneficial in promoting healthy thyroid function due to copper, which aids the production and absorption of hormones. It has vitamin A that keeps the vision in good condition. It has more potassium than banana for the healthy heart rate and blood pressure. Because of the magnesium it relaxes the nerves and muscles. It helps treat constipation.

"Recent studies shows guava with skin increase 91% in sugar and 27% when peeled."

Brenda said, I recommend to you your family and friends without hesitation to snack on guava's.

"You may receive a survey in the mail. Please take a few minutes to fill it out."

"Papaya is one of the best fruits with a lot of health benefits, according to Brian. It is a natural medicine that cures many diseases infections and maintain good health. A cup of cubed papaya has 55 calories. Rich content in vitamin C, folate, vitamin A, vitamin E, fiber, and potassium. It has an orange hue when ripe. Green papaya helps in digestion and is use as a cold dish or cooking by Asians. Eating papaya almost to the point of spoilage and their vitamin A level increases and helps clear skin. It is high in fibers that lower the high cholesterol and support cardiovascular system. It gives a glowing skin and prevents against acne, pimples, skin and ear infections. It helps heal wounds and prevents blood clots. Papaya cures dengue. Prevents cataract formation. It helps protect against colon cancer. Helps nausea and constipation. Use for weight loss. Papaya maintains energy and vitality.

"The papaya leaf, tamarind, salt, with water is effective for menstrual pain. The seeds can kill ring worms inside your stomach.

"If you have latex allergy, you may be allergic to this food. *Glove users "LOOK OUT!"*

Brian said, "If I did not tell the truth they will take away my passport."

"Chickoo is a round or oval sweet fruit with a grainy texture. It has a sandy pale brown flesh a brown skin with a black shiny seeds. I suggest to open chickoo longitudinally. The tree grow in tropical climate and bear fruit after 5 years. The chickoo is a native to Mexico and brought to the Philippines during colonization.

"It is rich in fructose and sucrose. Rich in calories. It has vitamin A, vitamin C, vitamin E, iron, calcium, copper, phosphorous, magnesium, folate, potassium, rich in vitamin B group niacin, pyridoxine, thiamine, and riboflavin. It is rich in compound tannins, the polyphenolic antioxidants. It has an anti-inflamatory, anti-viral, anti-bacterial, anti-diarrheal, and anti-parasitic effects. It is good for gastritis, reflux esophagitis and hemorrhoids. It has a high energy content that fights fatigue and weakness. Chickoo is antispasmodic as it provides relief from pains and muscle spasm. The milky juice is effective in removing warts and fungal growth.

"To ripen chickoo fast put them in the bag of rice.

Just don't eat the skin and the black seeds," *Nitnit said, "I don't know what it is good for?"*

"I like jackfruit-the largest fruit in the world," Jino *said.* "It can weigh up to 80 pounds. It has a GI 16 and 95 calories. When young could be used in vegetable. A ripened jackfruit is soft yellowish edible bulbs and have a delicious sweet taste. It has vitamin C, rich in vitamin B6, folic acid, high in fibers and water content, potassium, magnesium and manganese. The fruit is also used in jam, jelly, and addition to fruit salad. It is beneficial to asthma, anemia, cancer, maintains blood pressure and prevents constipation.

"Consider applying little coconut oil on the hands to solve latex benign catastrophe.

The jackfruit seeds could be boiled or roasted and eaten. It is rich in fiber, vitamin A, vitamin C, vitamin B, calcium, and phosphorous. Health benefits for the seeds are numerous. Food for hair growth and prevents hair loss. Prevents dry and brittle hair. Good for indigestion. Anti-ulcer and anti hypertensive."

Jino said, "Jackfruit is jack of all fruits!"

*"**Lanzones** originally from Malaysia and they call this fruit langsat. It grows across Asia from India, Indonesia, Thailand and to the Philippines. Lanzones has myriad health benefits. It is rich in protein, calcium, phosphorous, vitamin A, vitamin C(ascorbic acid) vitamin B1(thiamin), vitamin B2(riboflavin), vitamin E, minerals, and antioxidant protecting cells from free radicals associated with medical diseases. It prevents colon cancer. Powdered seeds are used to reduce fever. The fruit peel is dried and burned to repel mosquitos and used to intestinal parasites and diarrhea."*

"You can only use your hands to open them and eat. One of the healthy season's treat," according to Berenice.

"I like *star apple known also as caimito,*" said. *Geraldine.* "It is an exotic sweet tropical fruit that has 67 calories in a cup. Named for its star like design when sliced. A Spanish explorer Cieza de Leon who discovered it growing in Peru and made its way to the Philippines, Panama, Argentina, Carribean Islands, India and later the United States in Florida, and Hawaii. The skin is inedible dark-purple, with dark purple pulp or pale green with a milky white pulp. The pulp is glossy, milky, smooth and leathery. It is source of calcium, vitamin C, vitamin A, iron, fiber, protein and potassium.

"Believed to help diabetes, cancer and rheumatoid arthritis.

"Excess of consumption can cause constipation.

"Ripe fruit remain in good condition for three weeks."

"As best as I know *raisins*, are sweet treat that won't cause cavities and make you happy. It slows the growth of bacteria for tooth decay and gum disease," said Nardo.

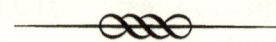

"Do you know that *Dates* contain more potassium than bananas?" Auntie Puring said, as best as I know...

"It is cholesterol, fat, and sodium free."

"It has calcium, copper, iron, magnesium, vitamin A, vitamin C, vitamin B1, vitamin B2, vitamin B3(niacin), vitamin B5, fiber, mineral and phosphorous.

"Only five Dates daily is necessary for a balanced and healthy diet will meet your goal for fruit. It has more calories than most fruits.

"It is a remedy for alcohol intoxication, abdominal cancer, constipation, heart problem, intestinal disorder, and sexual weakness.

"It helps diabetes elevated blood glucose by decreasing levels. Also helps lower the cholesterol levels especially LDL. It helps control heart rate and blood pressure.

"Dried dates keep up to a year in the refrigerator. If stored in the kitchen cabinet for a month they will stay fresh."

"I like *coconut*," Ben said.

"Among Asians it is called the Tree of Life. Both a source of the food and medicine.

"Green coconut are young found more in tropical places has a very soft meat inside and a sweet coconut milk.

"It has a lesser calories than any other oil. The fat content converted into energy does not lead to accumulation of fat in the heart and arteries. It is rich in fiber, vitamins, and mineral.

"It is antibacterial, antifungal, and antiviral.

"It gives you strength to walk the plank.

"It helps control blood sugar and improves secretion of insulin. Effective in abscesses, asthma, baldness, bronchitis, bruises, burns, gingivitis, gonorrhea, irregular and painful menstruation, jaundice, kidney stones, lice, nausea, rash, scabies, shiny hair, skin infection, stress, sore throat, swelling, syphilis, toothache, tuberculosis, upset stomach, weakness, and speeds up wound healing process far beyond that of any other dietary oil.

It is the **HEALTHIEST OIL ON EARTH.**"

"I like *onion*," said Manny. "It is rich in biotin, manganese, vitamin B2, vitamin B6, vitamin C, copper, fibers(part of grains before they are processed) phosphorous, folate and chromium. Chromium is a mineral that helps cells respond to insulin, that assist with blood glucose control. Green onions, because of their green tops, rich source of vitamin A. Onion increases HDL cholesterol especially when eaten raw. It helps decrease LDL or bad cholesterol and increase ability to dissolve blood clots. Excellent antioxidant(helps repair cells and may reduce the effect of aging), flavonoids, fighting cancer and fighting bacteria. When consumed daily if you have infection it heals faster and it protects you from getting sick.

"Ooops! Just don't eat onion before an important date."

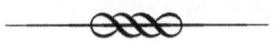

"Garlic is used as flavoring in cooking and used as medicine to prevent and treat wide range of many conditions and diseases throughout ancient and modern history.

"½ to 1 clove of *garlic* daily reduces cholesterol, LDL(bad cholesterol) raises HDL(good cholesterol) in the bloodstream. Reduces risk of stomach, breast, lung, prostate, rectal, colon and esophageal cancer. It lowers blood pressure and decreases blood clots developing. It fights atherosclerosis(hardening of the artery), bronchitis, tuberculosis, rheumatism, diabetes, dysentery, colic, flatulence, intestinal worms, ringworm, athletes foot and fever. It fights viruses and bacteria therefore helps prevent infection.

"Do not cook garlic at high temperatures or too long as it will destroy the compound known as "alicin" that makes garlic a healing nature.

"It would be real expensive drug if garlic is produced in the laboratory," according to Belen V.

"Go for the red when choosing for *cabbage*-it contains more protective phytonutrients and antioxidant. One cup of raw shredded carbohydrate provide 34% recommended vitamin C for adult. Cabbage contains soluble and insoluble fibers and soluble lower risk of diabetes and high blood cholesterol. Abundant in vitamin C, which supports a healthy immune system, decreases blood pressure, heart disease, cancer and osteoarthritis.

"Cabbage raw and short-cooked, show cancer-preventive benefits while long cooked cabbage has no benefits. Steaming is a better way to take advantage of glucosinolates(natural components of pungent plant) found in cabbage. The pungency are due to mustard oil produced from glucosinolates when the plant is chewed. Other method of cabbage destroys myrosinase enzymes, to help convert glucosinolates into cancer-preventive compounds. Cabbage can lower cholesterol if cooked by steaming. The fiber related components in cabbage bind together bile acids when they've been steamed.

"Cabbage will last two to three times longer as long as any other vegetables in the fridge," according to Auntie Inday.

"Broccoli considered a superfood for its disease-fighting properties. Rich in high fiber, antioxidant, beta-carotene, vitamin B6, vitamin C, folate, and the flavonoid kaempferol that fight infection. Broccoli contains sulforaphane that helps cleanse cancer causing compounds in the body. Rats were given sulforaphane lowered their blood pressure and improved kidney function. Helps macular degeneration, cataract and fight vision loss because it contains lutein. It slows or combat osteoarthritis. May have some protection against heart disease and stroke because of glucoraphanin nutrient. It reduces blood sugar levels as it contains soluble fiber and chromium," according to Elizur.

"I like *eggplant*," Britt said. "It is long deep purple, glossy and has a spongy texture and unique taste. Eggplant grow hanging from the vines of a plant. It is low GI, photonutrients, antioxidant, anti cancer, antimicrobial, and antiviral. One cup has 35 calories. It is rich in fiber, copper, manganese, potassium, folate, niacin, iron, calcium, vitamin B1, vitamin B3, vitamin B6, vitamin C, mineral, and vitamin K. High in bioflavonoids controls high blood pressure, lowers blood cholesterol and relieve stress. In the eggplant smooth shiny skin is nasunin a potent antioxidant and block free radical attack to protect cell membranes.

"Today the leading growers of eggplant are ITALY, TURKEY, CHINA, EGYPT, and JAPAN.

Avoid purchasing eggplant that has been waxed.

Oops... Don't char the skin and throw it away."

"Hey, *Spinach* is top for me," said Nenette Jackson. "It has 41 calories per cup and very low GI. It has an antioxidant protection, anti-inflammatory, benefit against oxidative stress related-problems, bone, cancers, and cardiovascular effect. It has an excellent vitamin K, vitamin A, vitamin C, manganese, folate, magnesium, copper, vitamin B2, vitamin B6, vitamin E, calcium, potassium and fiber. With it's high calcium content, it helps thicken and strengthen nails. It helps hair follicles produce sebum that adds shine and prevent dry, brittle hair.

"Individuals with kidney stones and gout limit your intake.

"Because of it's acid contents do not cover the pot when cooking and discard boiling water after cooking. Boiling spinach helps decrease the oxalate acid by as much as 50%. Oxalate is a compound that is naturally present in many foods and spinach is known to increase oxalate in the urine. Do not drink the water or use it for stock."

"One of my favorite perennial vegetables is *asparagus*," Belle said. "It is very low GI and eight medium-sized is 25 calories. It is good source of potassium, folic acid, copper, vitamin B1, vitamin B2, vitamin B6, vitamin A, vitamin C, vitamin E, vitamin K, fiber, folacin, magnesium, iron chromium, mineral and protein. One of the richest sources of rutin, a compound which strengthens capillary walls. It is low in sodium. It enhances ability of insulin to transport glucose from the bloodstream into cells. Vitamin A is essential to the maintenance and repair of healthy skin. Asparagus contain saponins that have shown anti-inflammatory, anti-cancer, control of blood sugar, and control of blood fat levels. May help slow down aging process.

"It can be cooked in many ways or enjoyed raw. Grill stir- fry or roast asparagus will preserve the nutritional value and content.

"Asparagus contain compound that when metabolized gives the smell in the urine. You are not in danger from eating this vegetable even with the strong odor urine. Pssst, the younger the asparagus the stronger the odor."

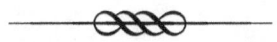

"I like *okra*," Meg Esther said. "The plant is cultivated in warm weather around the world. Okra plants bears edible green colored pods and it takes about 45 – 60 days to harvest. It has a small round white colored seeds. The pods are handpicked but you may use gloves to prevent tiny spines that might irritate your skin. No irritation whatsoever when you eat them. There is a slime characteristic when okra is cooked.

"It is rich in vitamin A, high in vitamin C, vitamin K, folate, vitamin B6, beta carotene, source of high fiber soluble and insoluble. Good source of calcium, manganese, magnesium, and potassium. It is very low calorie vegetable. It stabilizes blood sugar and helps control rate at which sugar is absorbed. Promotes healthy pregnancy by helping a woman's risk of having a child with a brain or spinal cord effect. Helps reduced kidney damage. Promotes healing process of cuts and wounds. Gives relief from respiratory distress like asthma."

Meg said, "I don't see any reason why anyone won't eat okra with all the health benefits."

"China the greatest growers of *sweet potatoes* and in United States grown from Southern States. Brought to the Philippines in 16th century by Spanish explorers and to Africa, India and Indonesia," according to Auntie Edith.

"Sweet potatoes can be orange, yellow, white, and purple. Rich in vitamin A, medium glycemic index, with 180 calories for one medium size. By boiling and roasting have shown better blood sugar result. The storage protein called sporamin helps prevent oxidative damage to the cells, brain, nerve tissue, throughout the body. How sweet it is to eat potatoes to reduce all inflammations.

"Vegan's, "LET THE SUNSHINE IN," Jovian said. *"IF NOT, A SUPPLEMENT MAY BE NECESSARY."*

"My passion for natural health drives me to tell you" Dr. Nelson Flotilde said, "**Make habitual consumption of nut to prevent cardiovascular disease and increase life expectancy." Overall, those who eat nuts daily have 20% reduction in death from all causes and 29% in death from heart disease.**

"When not to go nuts," Millet Mariano said, "can elevate both your blood pressure and your dress size.

"In order to get a **"desired dose"** from the nuts, experiment eating nuts, and observe how your body respond," Shem said.

"Just how much nuts you should eat?

"You mean my personal opinion? One ounce of nuts (handful) five times per week is enough," said Daisy Sulit.

"Something is up, uh, you know accu-chek **READING** down there.

"GO NUTS"

"Macademia nuts considered the world's finest nuts," Arthur Adan said. "Australia is the largest producer of macademia nuts. It is rich in vitamin A, iron, protein, thiamin, revoflavin, niacin, folates, potassium, phosphorous, and magnesium. It is high in saturated fats that lower cholesterol triglycerides and reduces risk of cardiovascular disease. Because of monounsaturated fats it promotes weight loss. Iron required for red blood cell formation. The fatty acids make them satisfying food and helps curb the appetite. It's omega 3 content prevents arthritis and osteoporosis.

"Pistacios are rich in fiber, copper, vitamin B6, potassium, phosphorous, manganese, magnesium, decrease LDL levels and antioxidants. Copper is necessary for iron absorption. Manganese is necessary for bone formation. It promotes blood production of the red blood cells, lowers blood pressure, protects the eye, strengthens immune system that makes your body fit, as best as I know Edgar said.

"Pine nuts have more protein than any nut or seed and are packed with vitamin A, vitamin C, and vitamin D," Joshua said."DON'T LET THEIR SMALL SIZE FOOL YOU."

"Hazelnuts has the highest folate and proanthocyandin contents that any tree nuts. It is low in saturated fat, rich in protein, contains vitamin E, high in B vitamins B2, B3, B5, B9, biotin, that promotes healthy skin and hair. The B vitamins prevents stress, anxiety, depression and improves memory. It improves healthy red blood cells. Helps reduce the risk of blood clotting and urinary tract infection due to proanthocyandin content. It's vitamin E, helps protect skin from skin cancer and premature aging. It encourages muscle contraction and helps muscle to relax. This prevents soreness, spasm, cramps, muscle tension, and fatigue. It increased the strength of the muscle the higher the magnesium level. According to Lina Litogot, "Turkey is the largest producer of hazelnuts in the world with 75% of worldwide production."

Joneflor said, *"brazil nuts is three sided shape with sweet nutty flavor and white meat. The tree has 500-700 years of lifespan and grow in Brazil, Bolivia, and Peru. Bolivia is the greatest exporter of the brazil nuts.* It has more selenium to protect prostate cancer, prevents coronary artery and liver disease. It helps support immunity and heal wound. You only need three brazil nuts to get the required selenium a day.

"Walnuts have the highest level of polyphenolic antioxidants(prevents certain disease mechanism from occurring) *than any* nut*s.* It provides a rich supply of omega-3 fatty acid. Handful of walnuts contains almost as much omega-3 fatty acid as 3 ounces of salmon. Eating 6-7 average size walnut a day could help scavenge disease. Rich source of energy. It dissolves blood clots and protects against heart arrhythmia. Prevents arthritis and depression. It improves memory and protects brain functioning decline that occurs with aging," Jovian said.

"Make *almonds* a staple in your healthy daily way of eating" Maria Luisa Hakuta, said. "When purchasing make sure no sugar, corn syrup, other ingredients, or preservatives have been added.

"Almonds are rich in fiber, potassium, copper, vitamins E, B2, manganese, magnesium, high in monounsaturated fats to reduce heart disease.

"Almonds decrease after-meal rises in blood sugar. It helps prevent gallstones. Protects against high blood pressure and atherosclerosis. It strengthens nerves and tones the muscles. Helps overcome stress, depression and fatigue.

Snacking on almonds will reduce your hunger and satiating effect helping you feel full longer.

Almonds can reduce cholesterol levels, it can reduce C-reactive protein, a marker of artery-damaging inflammation as much as first generation statin drugs."

"*Cashew* has hi fiber protein is low in unsaturated fat and monounsaturated fat. When monounsaturated fat added to low-fat diet can help reduce triglyceride levels. Cashew nut considered to be low–fat nut. High triglyceride levels increased risk for heart disease. There are myriad beneficial effects. It kills bacteria, reduces fever, blood sugar, stops loose stool, drying secretions, and reduces gallstone disease. Nigeria is the largest producing country of cashews. Eat cashews especially for people with diabetes, remember it reduces glucose level," according to Ben.

"*Chestnut* is low in fat and the *only nut that contain vitamin C*," Jenny Vi said, as best as I know.

Bess said, "I have some good recipes that are sure to drive you nuts.

"*You are suppose to laugh*"

"How much fiber do you get in your diet?"

- Alessandro said, "My meals mostly provide fiber, whole grains, (seeds from plants) vegetables, and fruits on regular basis. I have at least one serving of fruit and vegetable every meal. I try to select snacks that will supply what I am missing for a healthy diet."

- Fe said, "I like to fine-tune my diet. I tend to eat what's available but probably not enough as I should. I have cut vegetables in the refrigerator where they're easy to grab and within reach. I eat lots of polyunsaturated fats found in nuts and seeds. I know which food to eat more and which food to limit so I am on my way to heart healthy diet."

- "Guess what? I'm learning to manage this type 2 diabetes. I'm making some simple lifestyle changes that I can enjoy and stay with. I eat lots of vitamin A that include dark green and yellow vegetables and fruits i.e. carrots, sweet potato, pumpkin, squash, broccoli, spinach, turnip, greens, kale, sweet peppers, apricot and cantaloupe. This will help protect against the complications of diabetes such as retina and kidney problems. I'm on a groundbreaking eating plan eating well-balanced meals in the correct amount to manage the blood sugar levels and reverse this chronic disease," Catalina said.

- "My diet consists of whole grains, legumes, fresh fruits, vegetables, lean meat and food lower in fat and sugar," said Gary. I treat snack time like mealtime varying choices from among the healthy servings of protein and fibers. I exercise religiously."

- "Shh," Antonio said, "I focus on restoring concentration between meals. Nuts, dried fruits, fresh fruits, low fat cheese, and low fat yogurt. I eat fruits and vegetables and only lean meat. I drink plenty of water every single day. For change sometimes I add cucumber or citrus slices to my water. Hydration is key to felling your best."

- "Look!" Emilio said. "I am high on green leafy vegetables but moderate on fruits and meat. I choose wisely on healthful snack options staying away candies, chips, cookies and soda which negatively impact health."

- Rowena said, "I followed Vegan diet. I eat entirely plant-based diet with lots of fruits, vegetables, whole grain, and no animal products. I like cucumber it is the lowest calorie vegetables that provide valuable antioxidant, anti-inflammatory and anti cancer benefits. It cleanses and beautify the skin. I aim for prevention of diabetes, weight loss, heart disease, and cancer."

- "I eat and watch TV all at the same time with my lean meat, veggies and fruits. I eat more low-calorie, nutrient-rich foods, and less high-calorie, less high-sodium food," claimed Ruth.

- "I aim for five to six small servings of meals per day. I eat foods, such as meats, sea foods, legumes, whole grains, nuts, and seeds. Zinc helps guard against infection. Fruits and vegetables are not good sources of zinc, but it is often part of my meal and I love to eat them," Myrna said.

- "It takes me twenty to thirty minutes to finish my meal," Liana said. "It is well-balanced healthy choices accompanied by veggies and fruits. I trim my fat off from meat for fats are high in calories. I often skip refined processed and fast foods."

- Chino said, "I like this deconstructed dish, fish and chips, with fruits and vegetables. I like apple the most popular fruits as it cleanse bowel, detoxify the liver and lower blood pressure. It is good for normal growth, development, and disease prevention. I eat variety of nuts and drink plenty of water."

- "Anywhere between twenty five to twenty minutes to eat my healthy diet with portion of veggies and fruits. I limit saturated and trans fat in my diet like butter, margarine and meat. I choose monounsaturated fats such as olive oil and canola oil," Kristina said.

- Janella said, "I am on a weight-loss program and follow a dietary plan. I include whole grains, seafood, vegetables, and fruits every meal."

- Neri said, "I exercise four to five days a week and follow a low-cholesterol low-fat and heart-healthy diet."

- Wally said, "I pay close attention in lowering my lipid levels. I consume diet rich in fiber like oatmeal fruits like apples, oranges, pears, vegetables like broccoli, brussels sprouts, beans, peas, soybeans, tofu, and soymilk. I choose wisely healthful snack options of nuts and seeds. I follow nutritious great tasting diet. I also exercise one hour every day. All regimens to return to normal state."

- Joe said, "I eat breakfast every day not to fall prey to viral infections. My morning food triple my body's interferon, a natural antiviral compound. I fill up on soluble fiber content of a bowl of oatmeal that can lower blood cholesterol and stabilizes blood glucose level. I include whole grains, nuts, vegetables, and fruits daily consumption for a wealth of health benefits. I love this recipe of saffron rice bright golden color that pleases my appetite. It has a delicate floral aroma and it is the most expensive spice. I take 3,000 ml of water daily because it is zero calorie. You don't have to search to stay hydrated. Drink water. It is good for digestion, circulating system, healthy skin, and brain functioning."

- Joseph asked, "WHAT'S FIBER?"

CHRONIC PASTRY TOXICITY FROM THE HOSPITAL BAKERY!!!!!

Romael Quirubin said, "When were done we don't want to leave."

"IT IS SHOCKINGLY GOOD!"

"I love dark chocolate," Nicah said. "It makes me smile, high in magnesium, mineral that calm muscles and relieve anxiety It contains anti-inflammatory compounds called flavonols that reduce both clotting and infection in the body."

"Want your smile longer? Auntie Bolit said, Eat salmon."

"What is the 'miracle' ingredient when boosting to your food's flavor?" Cayo asked.
"PORK LOVERS HAVE LONG KNOWN"

"Eat your Za'atar too." Serving Za'atar on bread is delicious simple food, simple enough to love it," Caesar said.
"It is a combination of ground dried oregano, ground sumac, marjoram, toasted sesame seeds, thyme, and may or may not add salt.
It is good for what ails you."

Selma said, "For those Health Foodies who jumped on every new food fad because it tastes good and healthy. *Clearing House Is Continually On The Move.*"

Ito Villagracia said, "There is a new fruit juice infused chocolate that has 50% less fat than the yesteryear. It is delicious with reduced guilt. **Chocoholics jump for joy!"**

"The results are more intriguing for *caffeinated beverages*! From coffee, tea, and soft drinks-increases energy and boost long-term memory," according to Colonel Antonio Funa, "DRINK UP!"

"I like *tea*," Von said.

"All tea is derived from a plant Carmellia Sinensis and includes black, green, white, and oolong. The difference between these types of tea is how the leaves are processed after picking.

"Green tea comes from the same plants as the black tea but twice more antioxidants than black tea because of the way the leaves are dried.

"Herbal tea is an infusion of different plants, flowers, herbs, barks, berries, fruits, and spices, and technically is not a tea.

"Tea bags offer convenience but the best quality tea is available in loose form. Loose tea is made up of leaves rather than powder. When tea leaves are broken up, that oil gives the flavor. Loose tea will unfurl when steeped in hot water.

"An average cup of tea has about 40 mg of caffeine and the highest is the black tea. Tea can be decaffeinated by rinsing the leaves about 20 seconds after initial brew.

"Tea's are full of catechins, antioxidant compounds that reduces artery plaque and infection. It helps lower blood pressure, prevents tooth decay, lower waist circumference, prevents cardiovascular disease, prevents cancer, lower Parkinson's disease, and acts as sunscreen. Every cup of tea reduces gum inflammation.

STEEPED, DITCH ME!"

"Lemon juice is good for you," said Cayo. "One cup is 25 calories can be used for weight loss. It is good for skin infection such as eczema. Add 8 drops of lemon to lukewarm water and one tablespoon of liquid honey soaked for 15 minutes 2-3 times a day, it will help counter the urge to scratch. The vitamin C is effective for glowing skin, helps fatigue, dizziness, tension and anxiety. The potassium content helps nourish the brain and nerve cells. Inhaling lemon helps concentration and alertness. Fights against eye problems and maintain healthy eyes. Lemon contains citric acid which prevents formation of wrinkles and effective in treating acne. It contains antibacterial properties that cleanses the liver, kidney, and strengthens immune system. For halitosis rinse mouth several times a day with squeezed lemon in lukewarm water. It helps reduce pain and inflammation in joints and knees as it dissolves uric acid. Beneficial for colon cancer because of it's pectin fiber. Aids in production of digestive juices and digestion and encourages production of bile.

"Soak cotton in lemon or spray into the air for insect repellant.

"The acidity of the lemon breaks down the fibers in the meat as a tenderizer.

"After consumption of lemon wait for half an hour before brushing your teeth to protect your teeth enamel."

"Drinking *red wine* prevents heart disease, stroke, anti cancer and anti-inflammatory. It can delay onset of aging and increase sharper minds because of the ingredient resveratrol found in grapes. Resveratrol-reduces melanin production by 50%.

"Caution, ideas on beefing up by imbibing more, did not provide more cognitive benefit. Excessive drinking can damage your liver and risk cancers such as throat and liver.

"A 4-ounces of glass of wine is equal to a 12-ounces of beer, or 1-ounce of liquor."

Belen V. said, "Drink one glass of wine, it works with fruit flies, fish, worm and YOU!"

Room 804 patient Arthur was so confused. He said, "the food that was chewed by others was given to him." The nurse Madol asked, "What did you have?" He answered, "Meatloaf!"

An 85-year-old woman has a new salt-free-diet order. After a few days of patiently consuming her meals, she told the nurse, "I am discovering more and more food I don't like," Lilia Henderin said.

Boyet was given broccoli soup. Then was asked by the nurse Daryl, "What did you just have?" Nonoy answered, "Now you are working again."

"Chicken soup supermarket brands prevented and alleviated my cold symptoms but my mother's chicken soup taste better." "That's the chicken story." Karl said.

The nurse Jovian Lily was asking a patient for a snack, "What do you drink? Apple, grape, cranberry, orange, pineapple, or water?" Emmanuel Pimentel answered, Aw shucks, "I want some GIN!"

Brian has been drinking milk and was asked if he would like more. He replied, "I want some afterwards."

"Doctor, you told me to stop drinking last month," said Bolot.
"Now you are telling me to drink one or two glasses a couple times a week. I am puzzled of the change of your plan."
The doctor said, "Research progresses tremendously."

95-year-old Peding was asked, "Where will he sit at the dinner table?" He answered, "Where the young ones are."

We have the best chef in the world in this hospital!
We have the best cook patient's!
We have a lot of questions and suggestions!!

A patient who was admitted in the psychiatric unit said, "I am being admitted because of consistent "humble pie," Shem Daniel said.

Another patient said, "I am admitted in this psychiatric department because of high pressure in my head?" Jershon Jeiel said.

"I was admitted in the psychiatric unit for evaluation because I like to talk. I was told I am hyperverbal. They set limits when I talk. Why do I have to lose my freedom of speech," said Jojo.

Jason said, "There is tsunami in me." Jovian asked, "Why?" He replied, "I'm in a mental hospital."

A manic-depressive Jared Ken went to see his psychiatrist. He told him, "Take off the pressure in me."

In the psychiatric floor, a patient said of her roommate, "She is irritable, anxious, nervous, restless, loud, and yelling constantly." Britt said, **"She is sick, and I am coping with her illness."**

"Outside my room there is a sign that says DO NOT DISTURB," Dodong said. "I need the sign that says, ALREADY DISTURBED ENTER WITH CAUTION."

He was admitted to the psychiatric unit for flashing residents at the nursing home. The nurse thinks he just needed a suspender.

Bessie sustained a fall before her admission into the hospital. A dry scab on the right forehead, the size of a quarter, is intact. Later that day she scratched her forehead, and it bleeds. She told the nurse, "The hard pillowcase injured my forehead."

"EQUALITY but let me come first. NURSE! NURSE! NURSE! NURSE! NURSE!"

Brenda was yelling repeatedly. Her voice could be heard in the patient's lounge, hall, visitor's waiting area, dining room, conference room, library, and nurse's station. The nurse asked, "Why are you yelling?" She answered, "To get the quickest attention and answer!"

Jovian, a nurse, reassured Tantan, a patient, "You are doing fine." Tantan said, "I am not doing fine. I don't know where I'm at."

Elizabeth Entero was admitted in the hospital because of not eating but drinking ensure and water.

Meals and snacks are offered many times throughout the day, but she continually refused solid food and continued taking liquids.

NEXT DAY SHE WAS SO CONFUSED THAT SHE TOOK THE TOAST.

Boday is always pacing. This morning she was anxious, restless, disoriented, pacing aimlessly in the hall. The nurse Shine said, "Why don't you have a sit and rest? You have been walking for a while." Boday said, **"I am not going to stop walking until I find my Doctor."**

Confused, disoriented, anxious, nervous, shaking, restless, fidgety, verbalizing, "Let me get out."

"Oh my gosh, where are you going Jovita Donato?"
"In the Emergency Room, it's full moon and Friday the 13th."

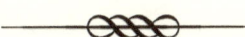

A 95-year-old Edwin was so confused and in the hospital. He was saying repeatedly, "I have to go to my car."

"Are you in a hurry to take your car out to escape high cost?"

"No, they have the best deal 15¢ per hour rate."

The nurse asked, "When was the last time you were in the hospital parking lot?"

Mario is unsteady and has a history of falls. He preferred to walk without assistance. Even though instruction and call light is given to him and he was told to call when ready to walk, he was not calling for assistance and continued attempting to walk alone.

Her daughter Joyce reminded him to put his call light on when wanting to get up still he does not use it.

For safety and to prevent more falls, a soft jacket restraint was placed on him and tied.

"Jeez! . . . Give me a break . . . ."

"I was born in Germany, and after I graduated, I went to Russia. I worked in the military for five years. I was a marine corps officer and an ex-navy seal. I have a good, memorable, and pleasant memory of that country."

"Oh, really?"

"Yes, really. I left my heart and legality.

"Oh, golly gee! Now I'm here in the hospital in United States of America, tied and locked in a civilian way."

The nurse is assisting a patient to bed and said, "I am helping you for the night." Camlon replied, "Yes, if you get on it."

Joshua was assisted to bed at bedtime by the nurse Shine. She raised both side rails up for safety.
When settled, he said, "Commander deposited forever."

Daryl, a nurse in the medical floor, woke Francis, a patient, to give his antibiotic medicine at four o'clock in the morning. After he woke up, he said, "Why did you wake me up? You are not an alarm clock."

"Do not take an illness that you can't afford." Bruce Wagner, said.
"Your insurance won't cover changing a battery in your pacemaker any longer. So, Tamar, here's the plan. From now on we will be giving you chest compression in the next several days."

Baden was rushed in the emergency room because of excruciating back pain. The nurse said, "I'm going to give you a bracelet with your name on it."
Baden asked, "Is it gold?"
"No," she replied.
"But it costs just as much."

The hospital is changing supplies to be cost-effective. Meg Esther is giving Dindin a toothbrush. Dindin said, "Microscopic toothbrush?"

A 15-year-old male Bert found in the room, trying to tie a bed sheet around his neck. Patient was tearful and sobbing. "I am sad and hopeless. I cannot endure this agonizing suffering for many things in my life are wrong."

He said, "Today is the day my brother died. He committed suicide. Why shouldn't I?"

"Why I am not successful?"

The bed sheet was confiscated by the staff. PRN medicine as ordered was given. Searched and clothing changed to scrubs with no drawstrings. Belongings and harmful items were taken and stored. He was informed to be with staff at all times until further order from the doctor. No discoloration noted, and the skin was intact. He was moved to a single room for suicide watch with continuous one to one care.

The staff expressed concern, support, and they acknowledged that his actions were caused by an illness and told that it can be treated and things will be better!

His good friends are in the waiting room and downstairs are Bebot, Panya, Paping, Randy, Bordigle, R-gee, Boy, Vivian, Julius, Julie Ann, Tomas, Victor, Nonoy, Bingbing, Roy, Regie, Jefferson, Ada, Joy, Janet, Elmer, Pagak, Marline, Tay Simo, Tay Mamer, Isming, Thelma, Totong, Balantito, Boloy, Edna, Elsa, Atang, Nating, Arlene, Roming, Igring, Oniok, Bonging, Aruk, Rusty and Raffy.

Iglesia, Ligaya, Oping, Soting, Antit, Aring and Arsing are in the cafeteria having snack. Joliet with her sister Alma Flotilde and Rhodora also with her younger sister Mabel Almanzor are in the hospital lobby.

The nurse whispered, "Msgr. Vicente Hilata is on his way to the hospital."

A worried Ken confronted his wife one night. "I have a problem with my judgment and a problem making decisions. I have a problem using the remote control of our TV. I lost interest in activities that were once enjoyable. I am lost in our house several times a day. I think I am in Italy, Holland, France, Greece, Sweden, Finland, Estonia, Bosnia, Poland, Ukraine, Austria, Spain, Switzerland, Ireland, Czech Republic, Norway, Hungary, Romania, Russia, Portugal, Kuwait, Saudi Arabia, Israel, Ethiopia, Nigeria, Ghana, Mexico, Colombia, Costa Rica, Puerto Rico, Venezuela, Australia, Singapore, Vietnam, Myanmar, Hong Kong, Indonesia, Korea, China, or Japan... Be glad that I am not speaking in Spanish. I have trouble remembering appointments, forget names…. misplace keys…. it keeps happening."

"I'm sorry, honey," Marilu, his wife, said. "This truly is a bummer to forget. The Doctor has to figure out what the problem is. Fix this—STAT."

"I have a memory problem," Joe A. Barrera said.
The doctor asked, "When did this problem start?"
Joe replied, "What problem?"

"Why are you here?" asked Elsa, the head nurse.
Evelio replied, "I sleep day and night and have nightmares while asleep. I don't have an appetite and don't know mealtimes consistently. I am too weak to even hold the phone. Ooh—it is heavy. Don't care to watch TV or read newspapers anymore. Can't get back to my bedroom, don't know where it is. Forgot my birthday and remembered after a week. Sometimes I could not remember a persons name. Short or over with day of the week or year. I would forget all kinds of things and my memory seemed to be getting pretty unreable. I am lonely, isolated, withdrawn, and sooooo sad."

Mira, a patient in the psychiatric floor, said, "You have *Alzheimer's and Depression.*"

"WE HAVE BEEN PROTOCOLED INTO OBLIVION." "ME? I'M THE KING OF THE WORLD." RICHARD LANGHORNE, SAID.

A 92-year-old man and a 90-year-old woman who were married were admitted in the hospital with Alzheimer's.

They were placed in the same room. Their beds were adjacent to each other.

The first night, he squeezed her hand and then turned over and went to sleep.

On the second night, the husband was reaching for his wife's hand, but she said, "Not tonight, dear. I have a headache . . . on Mondays."

The third night, the husband was reaching for his wife's hand, but she said, "Remember the doctor said I have bladder infection."

"I finally got my head together. Your body is falling apart."

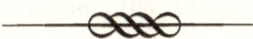

I was told by my doctor that I have depression.

He recommended ECT (electroconvulsive therapy) along with antidepressant medication and psychotherapy.

Nenette told her doctor, "You must treat this stress first for the stress you have created."

Jino was not eating but was drinking 7Up for three weeks.

His wife, Britta, took him to the hospital and was admitted to the psychiatric unit.

He was seen by the Psychiatrist. He recommended antidepressant medicine, psychotherapy, and to have ECT (electroconvulsive therapy).

After several ECT's, Jino started eating and drinking various kinds of liquids.

Daryl, the head nurse, asked, "How are you today?"

Jino answered,

"Yesterday I'm in and out of reality but today I have my full senses!"

Troy Lim, a patient in psychiatric floor was asked by Jovian Lily, the head nurse who said, "Yeah, are you going to join the group psychotherapy? It will start at 10 a.m. in the activity room."

"Well," he replied, I don't have to participate. **"I am the BOSS!"**

"If you're taking medication, make sure you take the right pill and right amount at the right time. Read the label two or more times. Don't double! It will give trouble!" Anna from Anna Maria Pasteria said.

"A medicine is that substance when swallowed, will produce a **medical report,"** Nelly Weiss said.

"The best vitamin for making friends is B1," Mary Aldousary said.

We like to save money. If it's inexpensive, it's not a bargain if it doesn't help you.
"Don't cheat your health with **cheap multivitamins,"** Jane Palomar said.

What is the *Vitamin that can boost moods, ward off depression and lower blood pressure?*
"It's vitamin D," Amparo Magno said.

Marilyn Villareal said, "I can take only original-brand drugs. I had rashes from *Generics*."

A doctor was writing a prescription. Nenita Roque said, *"I want to take one pill every four years."*

An old man accompanied by his wife went to see his Doctor. After the examination he was told to continue all his medications and add multivitamins one tablet every day. He could buy any brand from any drugstore where he wants to buy them. On their way home he asked, "Dearie, what multivitamin should I buy?" His 85-year-old wife replied, "VIAGRA!"

Dr. Vivian Barrera asked a nurse, "How was the patient that took twenty-two tablets of Tylenol yesterday?"

The nurse said, "Intubated in ICU, cold and clammy with missing temperature."

"The nurse is passing medicines in the psychiatric unit. After the nurse checked the wrist band of Patria Candel she said "please take your pills your doctor prescribed." She answered, "I will take the red white and blue you take the pink and yellow."

Prescy Kallansrude was telling Richard Kallansrude that the PRN medications are usually given on the initiative of the nurse. Nurses are often left to make the decision on when to administer a PRN along with what to give, how to give, and when to give. "Hmm," Richard said, "*This* is about to change dramatically. Have fun, enjoy, and be happy. REPEAT AS NECESSARY EVERY HOUR."

In the psychiatric floor, a man is isolative, withdrawn, and sleeping most of the time.

The Doctor told him and his wife to add new medicine for his treatment. "He should take *RITALIN* twice a day at eight o'clock in the morning and at noon. This would help his persistent pattern of inattention, help to improve symptoms as well as self-esteem, cognition, social and family interactions. Also it would increase wakefulness and increase focus and attention."

After a few days of taking the medicine on a daily basis, the wife was astounded with the progress. She began to notice that he is now staying mentally fit and focused. The patient improved and was discharged home.

One day, he was overcome with emotion at her sacrifice. "I want to thank you for all you did for me. *How can I repay you?"* She replied, *"Take that RITALIN 5:00 o'clock tonight*!"

Edith said, "Get a placebo, an inactive pharmaceutical substance given to compare the effect of the 'Real' treatment."

Brenda, Sandra, Canit, and Maya said in unison, "Spectacular, NO SIDE EFFECT!"

"Oh, golly," Edith said, **"This is the breakthrough, the PLACEBO has now side effects."**

"Vaccination is the most effective way to prevent flu," Gary Litogot said. "In the fall, you should receive the seasonal vaccine, although it may be taken throughout the flu season."

Lina said, "My doctor recommended that those at higher risk of complications from flu receive a flu shot. Pregnant women, adults age 65 and older, individuals of any age with chronic medical conditions such as asthma, diabetes, cancer and AIDS, healthcare workers who care for children and others."

Auntie Pilar said, "Stay away from those who are sneezing and coughing. When washing hands, use soap and water for 15 seconds before rinsing. Get 7-8 hours sleep, exercise regularly, eat healthy foods, manage stress and drink plenty of fluids. Know the symptoms of the flu: High fever over 100 degrees Fahrenheit, sore throat, congestion, cough, headaches, sudden onset of all-over body malaise, chills, loss of appetite, nausea, vomiting, fatigue and weakness. If you get sick, stay home avoid contact with family members. Seek medical care if you develop severe difficulty breathing too sick to do anything or if you cannot drink plenty of fluids."

It is hard to tell which made him miserable—taking the medicines by mouth or taking a rectal temperature?

Joneflor's guess is the rectal thermometer.

Do you wonder which drugs are invented, tested, approved, and released for medical purpose and use?

"TAP WATER ENEMA," Christopher said.

Bella said, "Some concept is important but needs instruction and warning. Like, for instance, increasing your fiber intake. Start with small amount and increase gradually in small amount. Give yourself a chance to adjust. Don't worry about side effects as they will decrease and eventually will go away. You will know if you are overdosing it if you have *Diarrhea*."

Guia asked Elmer if he had a bowel movement. He replied, "There's always a movement in there."

A patient complaining of constipation and no bowel movement when doctor's were making medical rounds at 8:00 AM.
The doctor asked, "When was the last time you went to the bathroom?" He replied, "I had good bowel movement yesterday but not today."
Have **"WE ONLY JUST BEGUN"**

A psychotic patient has a colostomy bag. She is anxious, restless, disoriented and confused. She uses very profane language and very loud. She pulled her colostomy bag, circling it in the air, saying, "The shit is flying."

"The 3rd most common cancer in the world is colorectal cancer. Screening and detecting cancers at earlier stage are more treatable and curable by 80-90%," according to Madge Gilroy.
"I do colonoscopy for a living, so be suspicious of the colonoscopy, consider some advice?"

"Nurse, I had an accident said, "Toto Bondo." I am sorry I can't help it, **Please laundry me."**

"*Wash your hands with soap and water* and scrub all surfaces for *15 seconds* before rinsing *to stop germs from spreading.* Good old soap and water help keep you and your family healthy. I encouraged regular hand washing before and after activities. Disinfecting cell phones, door knobs, light switches, surfaces you touch like tables, chairs, kitchen counters and other areas used for food preparation to stay healthy. Alcohol-based hand gel sanitizer for disinfection can be effective and are great use to your hand," said Pauline Roungchai.

The nurse was calling the dietary department because Samson changes his mind on the soup. The nurse said, "*MAKE THAT CHICKEN PEA.*"

Aquilina Funa yelled frantically, "Emergency, Emergency, Emergency, which way is the bathroom?" Ms Silva said, "Me too is looking for it."

"Do you have urinary incontinence when you cough, dance, exercise, heavy lift, laugh, run, sexual relationship or walk?" Ruben Hurtada asked?

"Yeah? Well . . . .? Overactive bladder is an involuntary contraction of the bladder muscle which means that your internal plumbing doesn't work the way it should be," Ramon Mestidio said.

"Urinary incontinence can be caused by infection," Maria said.

"95% of the time the cause of the incontinence is simply the price you pay for being a woman and having children," Celia Basamot said.

Erlinda Pericon said, "One out of every three women who have babies has incontinence."

"Incontinence is inherited. If the mother has it, all the daughters have it too," Thelma Odiaman, said.

Wilson Bernadas said, "Most people think that urinary incontinence is an "old woman's problem" but it is not true."

"I have an urgent and intense need to urinate and make frequent trips to the bathroom. It happens even after I emptied my bladder," Gerardo del Rosario said.

"I have to push in order to urinate. If I don't push when attempting to urinate then my urine just trickles out. I don't leak and wet my pant's," said Buenvenido Himan.

"Psssst" . . . . Minda Almanzor said, "I am voiding every half an hour without leaking."

Tarcila Bringuela said, "I have urinary urgency without leaking if I have to run quickly to the bathroom and have to break the bathroom door. **When the bathroom door is not broken I am leaking.**"

Berlita Booth said, "I wake up three to five times a night to go to urinate." Lilia Manua said, "your symptom is called nocturia."

"I sometimes do not completely empty my urine. It continues to leak after urinating said," Claudio Tapleras. "Your problem appears to be a post-micturation dribble," said Gaspar.

"I have an underactive bladder because I can hold more urine than normal. I cannot feel when the bladder is full, so I leak small amounts of urine as the bladder pressure builds," Nelson Fabiaña, said.

"I always rush to the bathroom. I assumed that the solution is to drink less fluid but my doctor told me if I drink less my urine becomes concentrated, which can irritate the bladder. Cutting back on fluids too much may make you run to the bathroom more, not less." Excelsa said.

Geronimo said, "I have a combination urge incontinence and stress incontinence." Edgardo Manua said, "Why don't you focus on dealing on the one that causes more of a problem. I heard exercise often helps with a stress type of bladder problem. Consult your doctor on what is best for you."

Ildefonso said, "You know that they sold more diapers for adults than babies."

Romeo Halang said, "I heard those people wear three pads per day and soaks through them and has worn them for many, many years before coming for medical intervention."

"My urinary incontinence solution is . . . Carmelito Tianchon said, *It is time to get treated to get the BEST BATHROOM!!*"

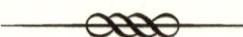

"I need a clean-catch urine sample from you" the nurse Sunshine said. "You wash your hands with soap and water. Dry your hands. Open the sterile specimen collection cup without touching the rim, inside the cup, or inner surface of the lid of the cup. Drink some water to help you urinate. Here is a water bottle" Glee said to Gabriel. "That won't help me I need a pop."

Brian could not urinate for eight hours. The male nurse said, "I will open the faucet and the shower. You will hear the sound of the water. That will help you stimulate to urinate. If you still can't urinate, I have to insert a foley catheter."

Brian said, "This is a catastrophic warfare."

Nong El has a foley catheter connected to the urinary bag. He is yelling loud, "Help! Help! Help! **"The urine is not moving. Call the plumber, I have a clog."**

Densiong a 92-year-old man, was disoriented and disrobes frequently. He took off his clothes especially when other patients were around.

One day Baden is in the patient's lounge, trying to urinate on the wall.

Densiong immediately took his shirt off and covered him.

"Hey, yeah," Baden said, "**Is this instant privacy?**"

Dr. Geordan asked, "Do you have a pain?"

The patient Meg answered, "I have a pain, pain, pain, pain."

I have a cold sores in prodrome and macular stage, Araceli Berano said. It is burning, tingling, focal itching, redness, and pain at the site where cold sores. Her son said, Lucky you, "You don't have a bump or blister."

Nitnit, a patient in the psychiatric floor, asked for a pain pill for her headache. On scale of 1 to 10, 1 is a little and 10 is worst. She said, "It's over 10." Nardo asked, "**Have you ever had 50?**"

"Most migraine patients are perfectly healthy between attacks! Patients almost never die from migraine."

"Put me on the list," Romeo Andrada said.

Manang is in the office for evaluation of pain. The Doctor said, "Please describe your pain after the fruit's name. Coconut for head, apple for knees, peaches for breasts, pears for back, pineapple for arms, and banana for legs. Where's your pain?"

"Mmmmm . . . FRUIT SALAD."

HOT or COLD COMFORT and SAFETY.

For chronic pain and stiffness at least 48 to 72 hours after injury apply hot treatment for 20 minutes 3x a day.

Sudden swelling from sprain, arthritis flare, muscle spasm apply cold treatment for 20 minutes 3x a day.

Do not use heat or cold treatment if you have an open wound, poor circulation, or if pain gets worse call your doctor, according to Botbot.

"Harold said, Test for cholesterol requires 12 hour's fasting before the test. Water is allowed.

A blood sample is taken from the vein.

Alter your diet with beer before test. NO TEST."

"Cholesterol is a soft, fat-like substance found in the bloodstream and in the body's cells. The body makes all the cholesterol it needs. The diet high in saturated fats, and trans fats you eat may cause additional cholesterol. In many cases, risks factor of high cholesterol levels are from unhealthy diet genetics and lack of exercise. When you have high cholesterol levels in your blood, it can join with fats and other substances to build up plaque in the inner walls of the arteries. The arteries can become clogged and narrow, and blood flow is reduced. If the plaque ruptures, a blood clot may form or a piece may break off and travel in the bloodstream. If a blood clot blocks the blood flow to your heart, it causes a heart attack. If a blood clot blocks the blood flow to your brain, it causes a stroke."

"How can I lower my bad cholesterol?" Elmer asked.

Harold answered, "Cut down on foods that include butter, cheese, whole-milk, egg yolks, shellfish, organ meats, fatty meats and other animal foods. Eat more fibers, fruits and vegetables, beans, whole grains, lean meats and poultry without skin, seafood with omega-3 acids, nuts like almond and walnuts, fortified yogurt, and olive oil. Exercise at least 30 minutes daily this will help increase HDL(good cholesterol). A higher level of HDL is associated with a lower risk of heart attacks. A normal HDL level for men is greater than 40 mg/dl. A normal HDL level for women is greater than 50 mg/dl. carries bad cholesterol away from the arteries and helps protect from heart attack and stroke. Lose weight if you need to."

Expedito Faciolan said, "A high level of LDL cholesterol in your bloodstream called "bad" cholesterol may raise your risk of heart attacks. Your LDL cholesterol should be less than 130 mg/dL but people with diabetes and cardiovascular disease is lower than 70mg/dL."

"The body converts excess alcohol. calories, and sugar into triglycerides, a type of fat that is carried in the blood. High triglycerides may risk heart disease. A normal triglycerides is less than 200 mg/dL," Gilda Entero said.

"Levels of creatinine indicate how well your kidney is working. The normal range is less than 1.3 mg/dL. If the level is elevated, it may mean the kidney is not working well," Anatita Biclar said.

"You look good. You are doing fine. Keep up the good work."
Because the result of your laboratory tests are so close to normal.
If any of your values are not in the normal range—it's abnormal.
Don't be cheated on this issue.
"GET A WIPEOUT," Nelsie Souchet said.

"I finally got my body together. Cholesterol, Bun, Creatinine, Albumin, Calcium, Glucose, and Uric acid all normal," Mr Lorenzo Lisbo said.
"Now I am nauseated and have a stomach ache."

"All reports are in," Delicia said, **"Life is now officially unfair."**

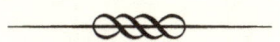

"Guess, who am I?" Nita said. "I am caused by buildup of monosodium urate crystal in the joint tendon and bursa. I can be a cause for long-term diuretic therapy for hypertension, use of certain medicine like aspirin, or a diet rich in protein.

"Usually I begin in the big toe, joint, followed in ankles, instep, knees, wrists, and elbows.

"I have an excess of uric acid in the blood and presence of such crystals in the joint fluid. This confirms the diagnosis of my disease. A risk factor of heart attack and stroke.

"My doctor gave me colchicine for the acute attacks and once acute symptoms have abated, recommended allopurinol."

Blessie said, "Are you a Goat?"

The normal medical student said, *"The correct answer is Gout."*

"Osteoporosis is thinning of bones—a decrease in the density of the bones."

"Concentrate on prevention because it has no trade-in value," Martin Funa said.

Risk Factors of Osteoporosis:

- Age 40 years or older
- Cigarette smoking
- Family members who have osteoporosis
- Heavy use of alcohol
- Lack of exercise
- Medical problems:
- Bronchitis
- Diabetes
- Emphysema
- Hyperthyroidism
- Injuries
- Low calcium
- Rheumatoid arthritis
- Medications: cortisone-like drugs
- Menopause
- Underweight

"Which people with risk factors will actually develop osteoporosis?"

"Osteoporosis has no known cure."

"It might live with you forever."

"RESEARCHERS caution to go Fast—FALLS MAY OCCUR IF YOU HURRY."

"I have headaches and abdominal pain. I have insomnia and fatigue. I am also sensitive to the texture of clothing. I went to see several specialists. They all run tests, but all show nothing wrong. My symptoms were decreased, but they did not treat my disease," Belen V. said.

"Once upon a time, I ran and jogged. I'm normal and happy. Now almost every few steps, I ache. I am irritable and can't get a good night's sleep. I had many diagnostic tests completed. I was told it's all in my head—that I need a psychiatrist," Jemima said.

"I have fatigue, exhaustion, and depression. My upper and lower knees and hips hurt. The pain feels like an ache. I made trips from clinic to clinic, hearing medical excuses. The good news was my tests were normal. The bad news was the doctors are not able to tell me what's wrong," Johana said.

"The magnificence of your existence knows no bounds! I spend most of my day in considerable pain and exhaustion. I have lumps and bumps. My fingernails are chipping. I find myself in frequent isolation, sad and depressed," Britta said.

"I may not seem like much fun to be with, but I'm more stuck inside a body with constant problem. I have leg cramps, muscle pain, stiffness, and lack of energy that I have little or no control. I am sensitive to stress. I go to bed in pain and wake up in pain. These doctors don't know that the pain is real," Jaclyn said.

"I called to make an appointment. My first was after I saw two different doctors. The receptionist with a foreign accent answered, but I could understand her well," according to Brenda.

"The day I have to see him, I am in modicum of apprehension. He introduced himself and asked me, to have a seat." Then he said, "How may I help you?" with a big smile, "but I like his tie."

"I had back pain, insomnia, and nervous legs with a whole awful feeling. He directed me to the room so he could examine me." "When did this all start?" I replied, "Two weeks ago."

We must run some tests, which was done afterwards. I was given prescriptions for pain, sleeping and nerve pills. He instructed me to return in seven days.

"I thanked him, smiled, and graciously left but was fixated on doom and gloom.

"I returned with my husband, Cayo; son, Von; and brother, Ben. That's a trifecta. I am nervous controlling myself to show good behavior.

I said, "The pain is slightly better, but my sleep is still poor and my legs are the same, nervous."

Seated in his cluttered desk, he said, "The test is back. Looks like the symptoms you manifested, the physical examination, and the laboratory test suggested most likely you have fibromyalgia."

Brenda said, "He was explaining my disease and the treatment plan for fifteen minutes. My ears are now troubling, and I can hear some. I pretended to understand them, but I did not. I wish he put it in writing and makes 12 copies. I hope my family listened attentively and heard every word he said as I am ready to make another appointment."

"I have fatigue, stiffness, and memory problems. So sensitive to smell and noises. I am so lucky I was diagnosed right away and treated correctly by Dr. Huinda," Enla said.

"I have fibromyalgia, and I learned a lot from him about my disease. I will forever be in his debt."

He said, "This disease knows no prevention. There are no geographic and racial boundaries. Women are predominantly more affected than men. Some young ones but average age on middle age. It is a genetic defect. It is caused by an abnormality in phosphate excretion."

I was given instructions to do active exercise on stretching and strengthening of the muscle involved and swimming.

I was taught the mind-body technique. To avoid negative thoughts with positive attitudes about life.

That memory and concentration impairment called fibro fog will go away once medicated.

I was told that nobody has died of fibromyalgia.

He told me to take Guaifenesin therapy for life.

Avoiding all sources of natural or synthetic salicylates. Strict adherence to the provided diet. A long list was given to me with every letter of the alphabet from A to Z is represented. To name a few, apricot, banana, capers, date, elderberry, fig, garlic, honey, thyme, vanilla, watermelon, and more.

He emphasized that Guaifenesin has no significant side effects and works only if you are taking your medicine. If you stop, Fibromyalgia returns.

Flare-ups and setbacks may occur. Re-alarm yourself to be in control. Learn the permanent restrictions and the coping skills.

I learned and practiced the mind-body treatment and it is rewarding. Now I sleep well at night and wake up in the morning refreshed. Not tired and my mental impairment went away.

The happiest of my life, "I am normal, the real me, and feel more than wonderful. I am amazed. All I hope is to live pain-free, and the good news is I don't have pain and that pessimism and low self-esteem is lifted with equanimous astonishing feeling."

"Let's see what the Twitter has to say."

There are numerous patients for admission in the hospital waiting area and are venting their symptoms.

Jovel said, "I have small red bumps and blisters on the side of the fingers, around the wrist, elbows, armpits, waists, thighs, nipples, breasts, and lower buttocks. It is itching particularly at night and a severe relentless itch." The doctor said, "I have Scabies."

Rene said, "I have, for several days, burning pain and sensitive skin. Then the rash starts as small blisters on a red base, with new blisters continuing to form. I have Shingles. You can only get shingles if you've had chickenpox. But if you never had chickenpox when the rash is blistering and you have a direct contact you can get chickenpox which later resurface as shingles."

"Oh my gosh, I have fever, headache, diarrhea, rose-colored spots on my trunk," Joseph said. "The doctor told me I have Typhoid Fever."

Lina said, "I have low-grade fever, chills, night sweats, fatigue, weight loss, persistent cough and coughing up mucus, wheezing and difficulty breathing. I cover my mouth every time I cough. I had a PPD skin test, sputum, blood test and chest X-ray." My doctor said, "I have Tuberculosis."

Fred said, "I have severe headache, painful stiff neck, high fever, nausea, vomiting, mottled skin, cold hand and feet, shivering, very sleepy and feeling unwell." The doctor just examined me and said, "The tests that were done—blood, spinal tap, X-ray, and scan—showed I have Meningitis."

Dax said, "Guess what? I have C-Diff. I think I got this from visiting a friend in the hospital."

"Hmm," Kiko mumbled, "from my last hospital admission I had MRSA. But I am staying up-to-date on vaccinations."

"What about me? I have MUMPS. Stiff neck and no appetite. I have swelling and tenderness in my jaw, mouth, and cheeks just below the front of my eyes," Tessa said.

Manang Bebe said, "I have infectious disease but not contagious."

Purificacion said, "I feel good. I don't have a symptom to be treated and ameliorated."

A retired Doctor told his good friend, Roman Schlaeger, about his newly diagnosed disease.

"Remember Dr. Hamid Hai? Very well indeed. One of the greatest doctors!"

"So as for you," the Doctor replied, "everything I see about you says you're one of the greatest architects!"

"Ahhhh, you know, I went to see him in the office as I am stiff in my body, arms, and legs. I am shaking in my hand and some tremors on one side of my body. My leg shakes when I sit down. I noticed the way I write letter sizes are smaller and the words crowd together. I have trouble smelling food. After thorough history and examination, he told me I have Parkinson's Disease."

You see, Parkinson's Disease is a chronic and progressive disorder of the nervous system. For some people the disease progresses quickly and others do not. It may ultimately become debilitating over a long time. In the brain there is a failure of the nerve cells to produce dopamine. When there is no dopamine, the brain is not able to transfer control movement. Therefore, there is involuntary movement and lack of movement.

It is named after James Parkinson, a physician from London, England who describe the "shaking palsy."

A soft smile played upon Roman's face, and he looked more sleepy than ever.

"Look," said the Doctor, "it was the worst day of this disease when I heard I have it. Since then it has been troubling me."

"Yes, Sir. It is a surefire way of setback."

"Ah, Sir!"

"Oh! certainly, The shock is not wearing off."

"Bothering strictly is the greatest concern," Roman pointed out.

"This is a serious undertaking. Give yourself what you can do, not one you can't."

"What do you have in mind?"

"Call Dr. Hai, EXCHANGE YOUR DISEASE."

"If you ever get sick, *CHOOSE A SICKNESS THAT HAS A CURE,"* Nena Tabobo said.

Teresita Florino, a 25-year-old female, went to neurologist because of her numbness of her entire left leg to the waist.
Thorough history, neurological examination, and MRI were done.
Found no abnormal findings.
The diagnosis written off was FALSE.

The most unpredictable of neurological disease is Multiple Sclerosis, "present today, gone tomorrow."
With first exacerbation, second, third attacks. What's next?
Long periods of remission.

"NO CASES OF PEOPLE RECORDED COMMITTED SUICIDE BECAUSE OF MULTIPLE SCLEROSIS," AMELIA MENDOZA SAID. "IT IS NOT A DISEASE WORTH LOSING OUR LIVES!"

Multiple Sclerosis is almost never a cause of death. Merle Fangco said, **"They can't get rid of me**."

"Diet, exercise, alcohol, not smoking, and stress in preventing stroke are things only you can control," Nene Victoria said.

Symptoms of stroke:

- Sudden confusion, trouble speaking or understanding
- Sudden seeing in one or both eyes
- Sudden trouble walking, dizziness, loss of balance or coordination
- Paralysis or numbness of face arm or leg

Consequences of stroke:

- Cognitive effects every day
- Crying or laughing uncontrollably
- Frustration and embarrassment

"BEAT it before it BEATS YOU."

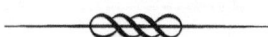

A middle age-Ben goes to a doctor for check-up.

The nurse Daryl said, "I have to draw blood for Hemoglobin A1C. This is your average daily sugar level reading in the past three months." "Helps check if your diabetes is in control.

"Ahh, I check my own blood sugar frequently. Ben said, I think the purpose of such testing is to increase paranoia.

The nurse said, **Justifiable Paranoia.**

So you've just been diagnosed with Type 2 DIABETES? The pancreas does not produce enough insulin or the cells fail to use the insulin the body produces. The glucose builds up resulting in high blood sugar.

It's resolution requires comprehensive approach. Education on self-care management is necessary in order to prevent complications like heart disease, cerebrovascular disease, kidney disease, retinopathy, nerve damage and foot problems. The health care involved in providing care should include the primary care physician, diabetes educator, dietitian, and support system.

Education should focus on healthy eating habits, blood glucose monitoring, exercise, medication, risks reduction, and healthy coping techniques.

The fastest growing lifestyle disease globally. Diabetes is not just all in your genes. Obesity and modern lifestyle are contributors. No one knows why people develop diabetes, but once diagnosed, you have it for life.

Aida said, "There is no one-size fits-all type of diabetic diet. Some respond to portion control and others carbohydrate counting meal planning."

"Eating white rice 5x or more increases type 2 diabetes by 17% and brown rice decrease by 11%. I like popcorn 31 calories per cup. I like brussels sprouts this low-carb vegetable is rich in fiber make me feel full without spiking blood sugar. Eat carrots to safeguard your eyes and immune system. Snack on fruits like guava, starfruit, black jamun, blueberries, strawberries, chickoo, cherries, peach, apple, pear, orange, and persimmon.

Remember carbs increase serotonin levels which can put you in a better mood and you "blew it" but be smart and realistic by drinking more water and by walking more. Monitor blood sugar, healthy eating and exercise regularly.

Hope this will help. Have a happy and long life!"

Guia said, "Type1 diabetes is failure of the body to produce insulin and requires the person to wear an insulin pump or inject insulin. Insulin pill or inhale puff does not work."

"I eat fiber-rich diet as it slows the absorption of carbohydrates avoids rapid increases in blood sugar levels and maybe even avoid-neuropathy."

Ben Hur said, "A natural way to fight diabetes-Boost Immunity and Slow Aging!" "If you are smoking-quit it can lead to heart attacks, stroke, kidney damage, foot amputation, and increases blood glucose reading. In exercise your body is using sugar to fuel the work of your muscles. Exercise effect lasts 12-14 hours and regular exercise offers longer-lasting benefits controlled blood sugar improved cholesterol levels and lower blood pressure. Exercise has been known to cause good health and happiness. Studies shows on whole grain eating reduces inflamation in diabetics. Keep blood pressure below 140/80 mmHg. To stabilize your sugar level is a trace element called chromium that is found in baked beans, peanut butter, shell fish, and whole grain. Vegan diet a diet that consumes vegetables, fruits, high fiber, low glycemic index food is strongly recommended. Refrain from animal products, keep oil low to tackle the problems. Apply lotion to your skin every night to keep skin moisturized to prevent cracking, peeling, and developing sores. Brush your teeth in the morning and at night, and floss every night. Get enough sleep as sleep deprive was linked to severe hypoglycemia risk."

"Remember you are responsible for the daily management of your diabetes.

"I strongly suggest to avoid going more than 5 hours without eating! "Do not skip a meal."

"Wear a medical alert bracelet." Ben said, "I liked my medical alert bracelet that I asked my jeweler to make me a matching earrings."

"If your blood sugar level is high 250mg/dl for two test in a row check your ketones in the urine. Do not exercise if your blood glucose is over 250mg/dl and ketones are present. Drink plenty of water to "wash out." There is not enough insulin to help your body use sugar for energy. Without enough insulin, the glucose builds up in the blood and makes the glucose high. Since the body is unable to use glucose for energy, it breaks down fat instead. When the body burns fat for energy, ketones form in the blood and spill into the urine. Symptoms of high levels of ketones: abdominal pain, confusion, dry cool skin, excessive thirst and urination, nausea and vomiting, and high blood sugar."

There are doctors and experts out there if you stay out of tract. Give them a Call for a solution and follow up with your healthcare team."

Symptoms of hyperglycemia or high blood glucose:

- blurred vision
- decreased healing
- drowsiness
- dry skin
- frequent thirst
- hunger
- frequent urination

If elevated blood glucose levels are untreated and continue to rise, the result can be HHNS (hyperosmolar hyperglycemia nonketotic syndrome) and, ultimately, death.

Symptoms of hypoglycemia or low blood glucose:

- hunger
- weakness
- fatigue
- fast heartbeat
- headache
- sweating
- dizziness
- anxious
- impaired vision
- irritability
- tremors
- coma

"Hypoglycemia is not to be taken lightly as it can happen at any time," Ben said. "Do you have something with you at all times in case your blood sugar gets low? Skip chocolate when you have low blood sugar. The fat in chocolate slows down your body's use of it's carbohydrate."

"Carry glucose source at all times. When impaired low occurs, you have available means to correct."

Even brief bouts of severe hypoglycemia can increase the risk of heart disease, Ann said.

Follow the "Rule of 15." Treat a blood glucose of 70mg/dl or less with:

- 15 grams of fast-acting carbohydrate like four glucose tablets, or half a cup of fruit juice, or half a cup of regular soda.
- After 15 minutes test blood glucose.
- If it's still too low, eat or drink another 15 grams of carbohydrate, wait 15 minutes, and retest as needed until your blood sugar is back to normal range.

"You can control it, don't let it control you." Ferdinand said, Lifetime modification. YOUR DESTINY is in YOUR HANDS!

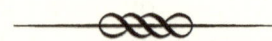

"Smoking is one of the greatest contributors to Heart Attack."

This risk factor does not require preparation for the test. "You know if you smoke."

A 100-year-old woman goes to see her doctor for physical checkup. She is alert, pleasant, not hard of hearing, neurologically intact, and ambulating well.

"Have you stopped smoking, Jennifer?"

"Ahh—Well, No."

The doctor asked, "What brand do you smoke?"

Martha Conrad said to John Ali, If you quit smoking there is no addiction development.

It lowers your chance of developing heart disease, emphysema and lung cancer

It helps you breathe easier

Increases your energy

Remember it saves you money and the inconvenience of the bad habit of smoking

If you quit smoking you can begin improving your health immediately."And it can add years to your life!"

Kathie Vinson said, "If you continue smoking cigarettes-increases your heart rate and blood pressure. It affects nearly every organ in your body and causes many diseases that reduces your health."

Betty asked, "Have you ever heard a doctor say not to quit smoking?"

Dany replied, "Not yet." "How about E–CIGS?" "No tar, toxic chemicals, smoke, smelly clothes, and you can smoke anywhere."

John asked, "Does St. Peter say that if you smoke, you can't get to heaven?"

Martha answered, "No, but the more you smoke, the sooner you'll get there."

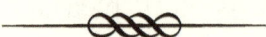

"What is high blood pressure?

"Blood pressure is the force of the blood pushing against the walls of the arteries. Your blood pressure is at its highest when the heart beats, pumping the blood *(systolic pressure)* and when the heart is at rest, the pressure is lower*(diastolic pressure). Blood pressure is provided in two numbers: systolic(top number) and diastolic(lower number) pressures and will appear one above the other such as 120/80.*

"A systolic blood pressure greater than 140 or diastolic blood pressure greater than 90 indicates high blood pressure or hypertension.

"High blood pressure increases the risk of coronary heart disease(which leads to heart attack) and stroke, especially along with other risk factors.

"If you have diabetes, gout, or kidney disease more likely you will have high blood pressure. You will more likely to develop high blood pressure if your parents have high blood pressure.

"Check with your doctor about or on the lifestyle changes that you can make to help lower your blood pressure."

"I have high blood pressure and my doctor adviced me on a healthy eating plan, more fruits, vegetables, whole grains, and less salt. A healthy diet low in total fat, saturated fat, and cholesterol. This will help me prevent stroke, heart attack, heart failure, and kidney failure," Baden said.

"My doctor told me the way to help my high blood pressure is lifestyle change and emphasize on lots of fruits, vegetables, whole grains, less saturated fat, low fat dairy products and no salt. Take the prescribed medicine and keep it at that level. Also I have to be more physically active with exercise 5 times a week. He does not know how and not to worry, just exercise even my knees are full of arthritis," Ben said.

Brenda said, "my doctor wants me to follow the Mediterranean style of eating to lower my blood pressure and protect against heart disease. To eat fruits, vegetables, whole grains, beans, legumes, nuts, herbs and spices. I have to use olive oil and not the other oils. Fish, poultry, eggs, and yogurt in moderate amounts. Red meat and sweets only occasionally. Red wine optional or moderation.

"Now I invested on organics and probiotics, I will see in my next visit what my doctor will say."

Inocencia Cayetano said, "Ankle brachial index is the ratio of the ankle systolic blood pressure to the arm systolic blood pressure, calculated separately for each leg. Values below 0.90 or above 1.40 are abnormal. This could be a leg artery blockage due to plaque builds up inside the artery."

"For many, the first symptom of Heart Disease is also the last!"

Don't be caught off guard. Know your risk now.
"Better late than never."

A little high in blood glucose
A little high in blood pressure
A little high in triglyceride
A little high in weight
A little low in HDL
I will worry a little.
"WORRY MUCH MORE!"

"How do I physically exercise my heart?"
"OPEN HEART," Janet Foucher, said.

"My doctor told me I have peripheral vascular disease," Nenette said. "What is that?" Bob asked.

Nenette answered, "It's often a narrowing of vessels that carry blood to the arms, stomach, kidneys and legs. There are two types:

"Functional PVDs the blood vessels are not physically damaged. These disease have symptoms of spasm that may come and go.

"Organic PVDs are caused by structural changes in the blood vessels like tissue damage and inflammation."

"Show your doctor your EYES. He can see what's going on in your BRAIN," Aurora Palomar, said.

"Brains are awesome. Yup . . .

"I wish everybody had one," Kristine Palomar Quirubin, said.

"Have you tried sneezing with your eyes open?" Rifat Syed asked.

"My wife says I never listen," Edgar said. "Yesterday my daughter told me the same, I never listen."

"Helloooooo! Did you hear me?"

No answer.

"Who listens?"

"The mind affects the skin. **Discontinue stress**. It can make you fall out," Eileen Palmes said.

"My doctor told me to avoid any unnecessary stress," Manoy said. "From now on I told my wife Tessie to open all the envelopes. Oops, I also log my moods on social media when I feel overwhelmed."

Mrs. Josefina Hiñola said, "Venting your feelings, fears, and frustrations and releasing those feelings by journaling nonstop writing and *NOT TO WORRY ON GRAMMAR AND SPELLING.*"

**"Socially connected predicts Greater Life Expectancy!
Education is associated with Longer Life Expectancy!**

*Phoebe Fangco said," "While waiting for a ride from
the doctor's office, talk to the person next to you, about
things that stress you out. Psst . . ."* Eleuterio Berano said,
"That's prolonging your lifespan."

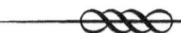

"I felt panicked, fearful, helpless, heartbroken, angry, frustrated, hurt, and shocked," Dodong said to Jo-Anne.

"Fasten your seat belt and that will make the ride less bumpy," Dennis said.

A retired schoolteacher, Brenda, developed redness and rashes all over her face and body.

She went to the dermatologist.

"Have you been treated for this rash before?" the Doctor asked.

"Yes, by my pharmacist, Edith."

"And what sort of foolish advice did she give you?"

"She recommended me to see you."

Jared told his Grandma, "Your face has wrinkles. I will help you straighten it out, and you will be beautiful." Grandma said, "How?" He answered, "I will get an iron."

"I'm losing 100 strands of hair every day. I'm hair-free by year's end," Nene said.

Nanay replied, "Iron found in eggs, helps with hair-loss prevention."

"How was your sleep?" Dr. Takao Ayabe asked.

Sharon Gardner replied, "What sleep?"

Prescy Kallansrude said, "getting enough sleep helps your immune system fight off whatever might be coming in you. (ick!)"

A 115 years old man, Tauro is in the hospital, telling his niece Brenda, "You know, my wife, Puring, has a beautiful heart like a bra and all the time in there for support."

"Nervous? Calm down, Keep smiling, give it a minute, and try over and over and over again, as best as I know" Rolando said.

What's Fatigue to You?

- Lack of energy and motivation
- Lethargy
- Pile of dirty pots, pans, and dishes
- Laundry pile
- Malaise
- Weary
- Tall grasses on my lawn
- Did you overwork or overplay?
- Did "Bacteria" stop by?
- Feeling rundown
- I'm exhausted
- Sooooo tired
- Weak
- Brain-fried
- Frazzled

"Universal fatigue? Nancy Roblete said, This will pass with BED REST!"

"Remember, when resting Canit said, RELAX!"

"Fatigue could affect anyone but if it becomes recurring problem," Nelton Fabiaña said, *"CONSULT YOUR DOCTOR!"*

Bess is animated; she said to the nurse Jovian, "Please give me red wine and light my cigarette."

The nurse asked, "Do you know where you are?"

The patient answered "no" shaking her head.

The nurse then said, "You are in the hospital and you came in yesterday morning with your son. Smoking is not permitted in the hospital, a rule that everyone abides of."

Bess became anxious, fidgety, enraged and yelled out loud. "Then, GIVE me BLOOD! GIVE me BLOOD! GIVE me BLOOD!"

Gilda Armonio said, "I will have surgery. My husband, son, and daughter all donated blood, but I need more."

Auntie Badit said, **"Yeah, all right, I like to stem your crisis. Is your pet a blood donor?"**

"Look!" a young intern said. "I have to draw blood gas to know your arterial oxygen." "I agreed even I don't like the needle stick."

"I don't see a coronary artery bypass grasp or a shunt in place. No history of cardiac catheterization via brachial route and no sclerotic vessels," the doctor said.

Richard Langhorn said, "I saw ice on emesis basin, prep kit, non-sterile and sterile gloves, needles, gauze, pre-heparinized syringe and band-aid.

He elevated slightly my head and turns my palm up. He put small rolled towel under my wrist.

He cleaned the skin with Betadine. Then he put on a pair of sterile gloves. Just trying to palpate your radial artery. I know this hurts, and may cause a burning sensation but try not to move. You will now get a needle stick. Stick, stick, ouch, stick, ouch, stick, ouch, ouch. It mitigated me, for he stopped."

"So sorry, I did not get it."

"I need the blood in artery that has oxygen in the lungs and is bright red." Moving to my right arm, he said, "I'm going to try this side. He enlists my cooperation in remaining still despite the discomfort until the procedure is completed. Prick, prick, prick, Oops . . . I have a venous blood. This isn't good. I have to try a different site. My apology this happened."

He put me in supine position and my legs straight. Again seeking an artery in the groin—again, again, and again and failed once again.

"Well! I still don't get it. I am really sorry. I will stop and let you rest for the moment. I will try again later."

Frequent trier—"NO!"

The surgeon and the nurse were scrubbing in preparation for heart surgery.

The nurse said, "Remember that midnight emergency heart transplant surgery?"

The doctor said, "Yeah, what about it?"

The nurse said, "You are not sterile."

What is a Doctor-Nurse Relationship? The Doctor is for the Nurse and the Nurse is for the Doctor. It's useless without the other!

"Patients make up their minds about their doctors within seconds after they meet," Ruel Magno said.

"So important to make good impression STAT!"

"So time is growing short. For your free-of-charge choice, to take your appendix out. Who could it be?" My psychiatrist, Karl answered.

Jojo said, "I have acne and want to see a doctor. **I wonder if the dermatologist fee is on sale?**"

The Radiologist is reading X-RAY films with the medical students. Dr. Lagunday says, "The patient has a great deal of pain in the knee because of the torn meniscus and ligament injury."

Then he asked the students, "What would you do in a case like this?"

The student said, "I suppose I will have a knee pain too."

Leonardo Vernell said, *"My hand has a fracture but is not broken."*

Dr. Vivian Barrera said, "I will listen to your lungs." (She lifted his shirt, and then placed the stethoscope on his back. She then asked him to breathe in and out through his mouth and listened carefully.)

Celso Cayetano said, *"I can only do this three times."*

The doctor said, "Open your mouth, I would like to see your throat. Say 'aah', 'aah', 'aah'.

Giovanni Borriello said, "This is tough to swallow, the tongue depressor smells like Popsicle?"

"What can you catch but not throw?" Von asked.
Jared replied, "You can catch and throw a cold."

JJ asked, "What is the one common thing shared by all four?
A person, dog, cave, and a river?"
Tantan said, **"MOUTH."**

Joshua asked, "What is the one common thing shared by all four?
A bottle, person, guitar, and river?"
Nicah said, **"NECK."**

Shem asked, "What is the one common thing shared by all four?
A pig, person, horse, and shoes?"
Nene said, **"FEET."**

Jov asked, "What is the one common thing shared by all four?
Siberian cat, valais sheep, person and komondor?"
Meg said, **"HAIR."**

Botbot asked, "What is the one common thing shared by all four?
Kingfisher, alligator, zebra, and person?"
Karl said, **"EYES."**

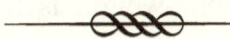

"Use small utensils that may dip your spoon rather than scoop. You will get better with practice and eventually, you will lose weight" Dindin said.

"If you're dieting, drink your milk and eat a low carbohydrate diet that is high in protein from dairy foods and exercise!
"People who lost weight while consuming protein with dairy products, no change in bone loss. People who lost weight while consuming protein without dairy foods showed bone loss," according to Dr. Beulah Roblete.

Chai said, "Give your intestine a workout." *Add some entries that require dynamic stretching workout for your jaw.*
"Remember your body would like you to EAT SLOWLY.
It is bad habit without breakfast, nighttime noshing on cookies and chips while watching television add to weight gain. You will eat less if you turn off the TV when you eat.
"Consider to brush your teeth early.
"The clean taste in your mouth will make you less likely to eat and you will lose weight."

"How much is too much?" Melvin Fabiaña asked.
Repeated, repeated, repeated colossal consumption. So "it is easy to determine the lethal dose," Jerry Biclar said.

"Aim for BMI (18.5 – 24.9); lose or gain if not there," Nad Mestidio said.
Ely Mendoza said, "Body Mass Index (BMI) is a way of looking at whether your weight is in the usual range for your height."

"If you are overweight, it is likely that you will have to buy some new clothes." Cancan said.
"Buy size 12, having to literally escape size 20.

"Can you think of any activity that is healthful?" Auntie Inday asked.

- Alleviates pain and improve body movement
- Better flexibility and strength
- Boosts energy
- Boost your good cholesterol, lowers your risk of stroke
- Controls blood pressure and decreases your risk of heart attack
- Decreases anxiety
- Decreases blood glucose and triglycerides
- Helps control weight

It maintains your trim profile
It makes your heart pump more efficiently
It strengthens your immune system

- It burns calories
- It increases bone density
- Increased endorphin level makes you euphoric
- Protect against hip fracture
- Physical activity is a true anti aging, anti diabetes elixir

Before starting, check with your doctor if you have limitations.

There's nothing to swallow and you choose your time.

"EXERCISE"

"For some people who do not enjoy traditional exercise there is a fun alternative for exercise, DANCE," Britt said.

"Dancing has a wide range of physical benefits in keeping us forever young.

"It improves cardiovascular fitness, and increases lung capacity.

"Dancing is a weight bearing activity that helps stronger bone endurance and aid in prevention of osteoporosis.

"Improves muscle strength and tone.

"Better balance that helps prevent fall.

"It reduces muscle aches.

"Dancing keep joints lubricated that helps prevent arthritis.

"It burns calories that helps control and decrease weight.

"It raises our good cholesterol(HDL) and lowers bad cholesterol(LDL).

"Dancing is good for diabetics as it helps lower blood sugar.

"Dancing improves our cognitive abilities by making us recall steps, styling, arm movement, turns and patterns.

"Dance and music bring people together in a fun environment and increases interaction thus prevents loneliness and isolation among seniors.

"Research shows that people who dance regularly have higher self-confidence and more positive outlook in life."

"Weight a Minute! I want to lose some weight," Onggong said. "I heard those who work out four times a week were 20% less likely to have a stroke than their couch-potatoe counterparts. A bonus benefit is to help prevent falls, and fend off-related injuries in case you tumble." Lewis Andrada said, "make your goal: 20 minutes a day 140 minutes of exercise a week!"

"How do you work out to burn belly fat?"

Elena Palonpon answered, "You can shed significant amount of body fat by doing sprint cycling for 20 minutes three times a week."

Bella said, "Weight is only a number and age is only a number." "I've decided that numbers are already starting to mess me up."

"How fit do you need to be?"

Gussie Mitchell answered, "How fit do you want to be, but in the shape to enjoy active lifestyle and reduce health conditions such as heart disease, diabetes and obesity, that regular exercise can prevent.

As you exercise to improve your fitness, remember that consistency is the key, your hard work will pay off."

"Are you all ready feet together knee's slightly bent stomach in and chest out, let's go." Dance the cha cha cha.....

Starting with the right foot 1, 2, 3, 4.
Okay, again starting with the right foot 1, 2, 3, 4.
Again starting with the right foot."
"Who did not find their right foot yet?"

"The count is 12, 13, 14 You have to smile"

"Some exercise is better than none, more exercise is generally good than less; No exercise can reach you soon at the end zone. Hydee Kramer said, *But resting usually feels better.*"

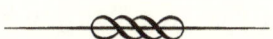

Lorna said, "Happy birthday, Edith. How old are you?"
"Oh, ummmmm, let's see," the lady pondered, "58 years."
"If you can't be honest, be vague."

"Happy birthday, Tony Boy. How old are you?"
"100 years old."
"Can you see me?"

"Happy birthday, Justin. How old are you?"
"102 years old."
"Can you hear me?"

"Happy birthday, Karl. How old are you?"
"105 years old."
"Can you still dance?"

"Happy birthday, Tantan. How old are you?"
"108 years old."
"Can you read?"

"Happy birthday, Jocelyn. How old are you?"
"I stop counting after I turned 50."

"Happy birthday, Von. How old are you?"
"120 years old."
"Do you still work on the computer?"

"Happy birthday, Jovian. How old are you?"
"124 years old."
"Can you touch your nose?"

"Happy birthday, Joshua. How old are you?"
"125 years old."
"Do you still play drums?"

"Happy birthday, JJ. How old are you?"
"130 years old"
"What day is today?"
"Monday"

"Happy birthday, Nene. How old are you?"
"134 years old"
"Do you still exercise?"
"Yes"

"Happy birthday, Meg. How old are you?"
"137 yrs old"
"Do you still dance?"
"Tomorrow"

"Happy birthday, Jared. How old are you?"
"138 years old."
"Can you walk?"
"Run"

"Happy birthday, Nicah. How old are you?"
"140 years old."
"Can you write your name?"
"Text"

"Happy birthday, Botbot. How old are you?"
"145 years old."
"Can you follow my finger?"
"Certainly"

"Happy birthday, Shem. How old are you?"
"150 years old"
"Do you remember me?"
"OF COURSE!"

"How can we tell how strong Shem is at 150 years?"

"UH-oh! Heard about the teabags?"

"You can't tell how strong it is until you put it in hot water."

"Ouch! Ouch! Ouch!"

Shem said, "I was in those disastrous experiences, I can take the next thing that comes along."

"Your name, Sir." The nurse asked.

"Brian."

"Your sex?"

"NO difference."

Posing said, "Don't worry about growing older. Older is better like vinegar."

Brenda asked, "Do you know your loooonnnnggggg options on *Osteoporosis*?"

"Hold it! Wait!" Ben said. Only the best treats will do for all of you. Let's move housewares for a grand party celebration.

"I understand your past and present, believe in your future.

"Even you are getting older I accept you all.

"To wish you Happy Birthday and then to tell you, too, There's nothing any nicer than remembering special you!

"My hug, kisses and wishing you all everything happy and joy on your birthday a day can bring and a very long healthy and quality of life!"

Veronica Leighton said, Here's your candles that sing. Make a wish before you extinguish in a single breath.

Katharine Martinez said, "God gave us the gift of life!"

Arnold Martinez said, "You have to accept whatever comes and be brave whatever you can. Love as many people as an option in life and here's your cake take a piece and only a piece."

Maria Fe Corpuz Bato said, "Hope you all have a terrific birthday and may this day be filled with love, joy and happiness.
"Let see that birthday smile!"

"Why are you giving me this document? What is this for?" Asked Ibrahim.

"This document is called Notice of Privacy Act." replied, Ahmed. Ibrahim, "But I want to be in the Facebook, Twitter, You Tube and App."

Ahmed: Want to do something fun?
Ibrahim: Echoed fun?
Ahmed: "May need to have those tonsils out."

"What is therapeutic lie?" Linda Storry answered, "GET A SECOND OPINION."

STOP THOSE LITTLE LIES everyday to boost your wellness.

Helene Para said. *"IT'S HONESTY THAT MAKES YOU HEALTHIER."*

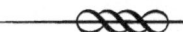

Fingernails grow two times faster than toe nails. Hazel said, "Mine is the opposite."

"You might want to double check on that?"

Cayo said, "I never make the same mistake twice." Von said, "he makes it 3-5 times just to be true."

Camlon said, "X-ray is a painless exam and nothing to swallow. It has a small dose of radiation to take pictures of the inside part of the body. "Gosh," the same day I have had a repeat chest X-ray."

Brenda ask, "Why?"

Camlon replied, "The technician said I held my breath two times longer."

"The heart CT scan is a test used to detect calcified plaque (calcium buildup) in the arteries that supply blood to the heart muscle (coronary arteries). There are certain types of soft plaque atherosclerosis that do not contain calcium build-up and cannot be seen on a CT scan. The amount of calcium in the coronary arteries reflects the total amount of atherosclerosis in these arteries and is a good predictor of heart problems. The score of zero coronary artery calcium is a low risk but does not mean there is no risk of heart attack," Marietta Fanco said.

"MRI (magnetic resonance imaging utilizes a powerful magnet and a computer to generate images). This procedure uses no radiation. It is capable of looking at how organs function.

"And when you are waiting for the doctor to give you the result of your MRI, seconds seems like an hour," Hya said.

"And when the result is NORMAL, an hour seems like a second," Harl said.

Two blondes talking:
"Listen, your hair looks like a wig."
"Truthfully it is a wig."
"Cool, it feels like a real hair."

"Did you ever have a chicken pox before?" Howard Lopez said "yes."
Rarely a second chicken pox does occur.
'Well you've got it again.'

"ALL THE BEST WITH HEALTH AND PROSPERITY," Nick Ovadias said.

"God loves us and loves to see us happy." Mary Slattery said.
"Wine?"
Estrella Daymiel ask, "What is the second choice?"

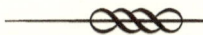

"There is a cute man sitting far right in the corner wearing a blue shirt. He is tall medium built and the expression of his face is happiness and contentment. He is looking and smiling at you constantly," Dawn said.

Ann replied, "It's hard to have privacy when you're in close quarters with many people in this waiting room. I get too fidgety to sit after a few minutes in a waiting room.

"If he wants a private conversation, he should make a sign or come to me. It never ceases to amaze me as I'm sitting that so many people you are going to meet."

The nurse said, "They are short-staffed and so they asked everyone to be patient."

Ann said, "I thought that's what I am, a patient."

"Shh, well," Dawn said to Ann.

"If he strikes a conversation, keep it brief and general as possible. Avoid going to clinical details."

The more "medical," the more serious you sound.

He might think of your problem as "TERMINAL ILLNESS."

Jeez . . . I have to say it is "toxic and hazardous while waiting, in this **"waiting room."**

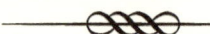

Eight patients and five relatives were waiting in the doctor's office.

There is always a waiting room that you have to sit in before you are seen by your doctor.

A flat screen TV is on and WiFi connection is visible. There is a big sign on top of the television: ATTENTION. Please Do Not Touch The Television. Thank You.

The magazines old and new are tidy on the rack. But it is shocking to see a daily newspaper subscription is available.

You are on time for your appointment, but your doctor seems to be running behind schedule sometimes.

The secretary comes out of the room and announces, "We thank you all for waiting, but the doctor won't be here for another hour. There is an emergency surgery that is going on that I regret to say. Again thank you for your patience. I appreciate your kind consideration on this matter and time."

Remember, there is no smoking in the office.
"Those pissed off about the One Hour Delay; please see the **nurse in the kitchen**."

Leonardo Sanders whispered to Don Russell, It's the perception of the wait that weighs and not the wait itself. Don R. replied, "Definitely!!!"
June Barrett asked how about something useful with their time telling them, "PIRACY CONTROL TECHNOLOGY and INDY BUILD?"

A big-eyed little old woman sad, tears coming down her cheek. She quietly bowed her head and knelt down. Her name is Rosario.

In the hospital chapel, I overheard her soft voice praying, Baden said.

"In my previous hospital admission I was near death but miraculously fully recovered. Hoping it's not long until I am well again." Wiping tears from her eyes again and again.

"I am praying that you will repeat that special treatment and care. Give me health, inner strength and come to my aid. Keep my eyes healthy. Enhance my hearing to listen to them. Boost my brain power and don't allow me to forget. May depression not find me. In this stressful moment give me a healthy doctor's report. I am hoping for the fast recovery and looking forward to be discharge from the hospital soon.

"Thank you for listening to me my God, and when responding please *"Speak Up Loud"* to my right ear."

"You know I love and enjoy my family and friends. I love to cook and bake. My regret is you did not try my signature hazelnut cake that everyone likes. The bark of my dog is music to me. That zumba, qi gong, tai chai, line dance, ballroom dancing, slide, and shuffle makes me happy and bright. I can dance and sing and loving everything. Smiling, laughing, having fun, and saying hi to everyone is delightful. My mailman brings me wonderful letters that fill my days with surprises and sunshine. I am a lover of nature and viewing many forms gives me happiness. My garden brings world of joys, totally ineffable that never end."

"I just want to stay much longer.
"I am not afraid to meet you, not really, really afraid. It is the other man I am afraid of."

An 80-year-old man, Tet was walking with his cane in the patient's lounge. A 92-year-old woman said, "I can hit him with that cane."

Visitors are sitting in the hospital lounge with plenty of doubts.

Brenda said, "I have noticed that all the Nurses check the expiration date of the medicines."

Bessie said, "Hey, yeah! I wonder if Dr. Rivera knows if a placebo has expiration." She added, "I better send him a text to find out."

Ben Hur said, "I most wonder if Dr. Obligacion checks zillion times their patient's lives—it has expiration date."

"Bring the MARINES! I'm ready to die," said the 100-year-old man. Virgilio Villagracia said, *"Don't forget to e-mail me your eternal address."*

A nice old man was telling his wife that if he died, he wanted her to promise to have his remains cremated. And the wife asked, "What do you want me to do with your ashes?" The man answered, "Flush me down in the toilet."

A doctor, a nurse, a transporter, and the CEO of a health insurance have all died.

At the gate, St. Peter asked, "What did you do?" The doctor answered, "I am a doctor. I apply medical knowledge and skills to the diagnosis, prevention and management of the diseases. I examined and treated thousands of patients who are suffering from diseases and injuries. I contributed to make them well to have their good health!"
St. Peter said, "That's great. Get inside the gate in to heaven. And tell me about you.

"I am a nurse. I took care of the sick and delivered an outstanding care regardless of religion, sex, cultural background, language, social standing, rich, or poor. I administered ease and alleviated pain of curing and treating patients' rapture of restored health. I help coordinate educating patients and relatives, engaging them to participate and follow their care plan. I offered advice and emotional support to patients their families and friends."
St. Peter said, "That's great! Get inside the gate in to heaven. And tell me about you."

"I am a transporter. I pick up and return patients to wherever their final destination may be. The operating room, echo lab, GI lab, physical therapy, eye clinic, stress test, x-ray department, and others."
St. Peter said, "That's great! Get inside the gate in to heaven. And tell me about you."

"I am the chairman of the board of a health insurance. I was in charge for the bills of their health care."

St. Peter said, "That's great! Get inside the gate in to heaven, but only for the weekend."

84 year old man came in for delirium changes in sensorium passing motion and incontinent of bladder and bowel two days prior to admission. Soiling himself and his room.

This morning while making rounds . . . . he said . . . . You are beautiful! . . . .

"Okay, the doctor with a big smile, said "I can discharge you now."

Andy is stable and plan to be discharged to an assisted-living facility. Arrangement was done by the social worker to the new place. Andy is well aware of it.

Tessie, the head nurse went into his room. "Oh, golly gee, ready to get out from the hospital? Where would be your new home?"

"Mmmm," he replied, "HERE."

Dr. Vivian Barrera said, "It's the day you have been waiting for—your ECT (electroconvulsive therapy) has ended. I bet you can't wait to get back to your 'real' life and put ECT behind you. A thought that comes to you on leaving the hospital, where you were watched closely, where everyone was focused on your getting well.

"Who will watch you now?"

Mary Slattery replied, "I applied for PLACEMENT in the hospital!"

John Ali went to the pharmacy to have prescription filled before being discharge from the hospital.

The pharmacy assistant Pong said, "How can I help you?"
"I wanna know if you have HCTZ."
"Well, this pill will treat blood pressure but does not cure it. It can help excessive fluid accumulation and swelling of the body. It can be used to treat kidney stones because it decreases the amount of calcium excreted by the kidneys in the urine. It will increase urination. It is a water pill," John said.

Editha, the pharmacist, overheard the question.
She suggested taking the medicine in the morning with or without food. This drug will make you drowsy so refrain from driving. Avoid exposure to sunlight. Wear protective sunglasses and sunscreen as it may make your skin sensitive to sunlight.

Call your doctor immediately if you experience of the following:

difficulty breathing and swallowing
bruising
skin rash
sore throat with fever

Call your doctor if any of these symptoms are severe or do not go away:

cramps
dizziness
diarrhea
headache
hair loss
thirst
muscle cramps

nausea
stomach pain

Include a low salt diet with potassium foods like bananas, prunes, raisins, and orange juice.

"The pharmacist said the medicine you want is—HYDROCHLOROTHIAZIDE."
"That's it! I can never remember that pill!"

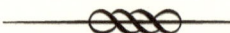

"The study doctor wants to know if I would like to be a part of a research genetics study," Antonio Funa said.

"My participation is voluntary."

"The nurse handed me a form which describes the study in detail and the doctor or the nurse will go over it in order to help me decide."

"There is a risk of confidentiality of information."

"In the event of an emergency, dial 911 immediately. If you require emergency care tell your provider of your participation in this study. Contact the study doctor or the study nurse as soon as possible."

"I will be paid for the time and participation for the study. I will not be paid extra for interim visits that may occur if it is necessary to repeat tests."

"The staff will take blood by sticking a needle in the arm. Drawing blood may result in pain, bleeding, bruising, irritation at the site of the needle stick and the possibility of infection."

"The blood will be used to look at the genes, which is called DNA."

"Genes are in our blood and they are what make you different from everyone else. Some genes might tell you about certain diseases, color of your eyes or hair."

"If you have questions ask the doctor about the study concerns or complaints and the consent form which was given to you."

"Being in the study will not help me receive any direct medical benefit. But I thought participating is my chance to give back what could help others and make a meaningful difference."

"Is there a guarantee against Alzheimer's Disease, Arthritis, Cancer, Dementia, Diabetes, Down Syndrome, Hearing and Vision Loss, Heart Disease, Hypertension, Muscular Dystrophy, Multiple Sclerosis, Parkinson's Disease, and Stroke?

"Your parent's pass on their genes. Your parents pass on Alzheimer, Cancer, Diabetes, Hemophilia, Ischemic Heart Disease, and Sickle Cell Disease.

"Your family helps define your health. The latter part of a life of a person is prone to have problems with various functions of the body. The cardiovascular, digestive, excretory, nervous, reproductive, and urinary systems are mostly affected.

"If they cannot harden they will wear out, Brenda Barrera said. They are a miserable set."

"It is not known whether human physical immortality is an achievable state.

"But perhaps a life full of longevity and the quantity and quality of life are achievable with technology, medical interventions, drugs, treatment, and cures of incurable diseases, exercising regularly, meditation, healthy lifestyle habits, good stress management, healthy diet (consuming a diet rich in vegetables, fruits, berries, onions, mushrooms, beans, nuts, seeds, whole grains and fish) and perhaps someday food technology and avoidance of tobacco.

"Increase in life expectancy with fountain of youth less money and suffering to beautiful years with family, friends, and strangers of the world.

"Live in tune with good health, physical, mental, emotional, and spiritual balance.

"Empower to Take Control, Logical Plan, Preventive Measures, Change to Healthy Diet and Therapeutic Lifestyle.

IT'S YOUR CALL!"

www.ingramcontent.com/pod-product-compliance
Lightning Source LLC
Chambersburg PA
CBHW021959170526
45157CB00003B/1062